"Ray gives us "shotgun" on this wife's fearless battle against CF. H his humor is refreshing, and his d Pay attention to his lessons in the . .... **Emily Schaller - Founder / CEO of Rock CF**

"Not just for Cystic Fibrosis, but for any loved one dealing with chronic illness - this is a must-read!!! Ray captures it all in this book... The ups and downs, the despair, the love, the absurdity, but mostly the resilience of the human spirit, to never give up in the face of overwhelming odds. To show that modern medical miracles are still possible. I can't recommend this book highly enough!!"
Ian Pettigrew - Photographer and Publisher

"Ray covers what cystic fibrosis is — how we take care of ourselves, our routines, our medications, trials and tribulations — the whole shebang…It is a great perspective reading about cystic fibrosis, a woman affected by it and having the proper support throughout that battle. I've lived through many of the events Rebecca experienced and I know just how important having a CF Cornerman is. It helps make your battle a WE thing, rather than a ME thing. Going into a fight for your life feels tipped in your favor with a great support system in play." **James Cameron – CF Trainer**

"The love and strength that comes through on the pages of *A CF Cornerman*, is unmistakable. The resilience of pushing to help those we love despite circumstances, through such a difficult journey to breathe and live is so powerful. This book is a must read to help show what true love is capable of when faced with the depths of hell. That becomes strength and pure happiness, from the love of a lifetime…a love we should all strive for."
Sandi Alvaro – CF Advocate and Blogger of *Behind the Smile of a Cystic*

Lessons from a CF Cornerman

38 Lessons I Learned During My Wife's Illness and Lung Transplant

RAYMOND L. POOLE

Photos © Raymond L. Poole

Some photos courtesy of Jessica Bastien, Melanie Romas, Rachel Saluzzi, Louise Poole, and Kate Bastien.

ISBN-13: 978-0692792100

DEDICATION

This book is dedicated to my wife Rebecca, a fighter with incredible strength.

CONTENTS

PREFACE

The lives of members of a Cystic Fibrosis (CF) family are hard, whether you are talking about the person who suffers from this debilitating disease or someone who simply supports a loved one in the fight. As the husband of a woman with CF, the coughing keeps me up at night, but I do not wake with a sore throat. I have to plan around the breathing treatments, but I do not have to do them. I'm worried during the ER visits, but I do not get poked with any needles. I spend hours in the hospital room, but I can leave to grab a snack. I do not have cystic fibrosis and I cannot take away her pain, so the best I can do is to support her and be in her corner.

My nearly thirty years of experience with martial arts has led to national championship matches, full contact bouts, and a focus on continual improvement. Throughout all of this, I learned that nobody can do it alone. I always had someone in my corner. Whether they were encouraging me, coaching me, or simply being present, their support was critical. A good cornerman offers tactical instruction, but more importantly, knows his fighter. He knows the fighter's strengths and weaknesses and how to motivate them to do their best. He looks at the fight from a unique perspective and helps the fighter refocus when necessary. But the one thing the cornerman cannot do is fight the fight for them. You dodge and move, get riled up, and suffer with every hit they receive, fully aware that they are the one taking every shot.

I wanted to write this book because I believe that the lessons I learned throughout my wife's battle with cystic fibrosis and her transplant journey can help others. It is meant for those who love and care for a person with CF and those who are care*givers*; those who fight

CF with the determined attitude that they are known for, those who fight any uphill battle when it comes to their health, and those who dedicate themselves to healthcare. This book is from my point of view, and like a cornerman watching his fighter face down an opponent, this perspective is unique. It is my hope that this book will provide valuable insights to those with any debilitating disease, their families, their friends, their medical team, and their caregivers.

INTRODUCTION

It was December 31, 2014, New Year's Eve morning, and I woke up with an optimistic attitude. I had completed the self-assessment portion of my job performance review the previous afternoon and rewarded myself with stellar marks. With a few days off for the holiday, I had the morning all to myself and planned to be productive. I was going to watch and delete several shows from our ever-growing DVR hard drive. I even planned to do some dishes while I watched. Maybe I would hit the gym then pack some supplies for our New Year's celebration in the hospital. Also, my wife was in the hospital.

It's not that I was unconcerned about her current situation, but we had dealt with this so many times before. Rebecca suffered from cystic fibrosis (CF), and when she started to feel sick, the standard treatment was hospitalization and intravenous (IV) antibiotics. This was so common for someone with CF that it was called a "tune-up." During the past few years, Becca was averaging two tune-ups per year. But 2014 had been a bit more challenging, and this was tune-up number six.

Rebecca was not rebounding as well as she used to, but that was the progressive nature of the disease. We also attributed some of it to the busy year we had—living apart for several months and ultimately moving to the greater Cincinnati area where I had accepted a new position. It seemed like she would bounce back as she always did, if she could just get a minute to rest. We knew that one day she would need a lung transplant, but that was probably not for another couple of years.

In the meantime, it was hard to break from our routine. We

both worked full time and made great money. In fact we both had more success in our careers than either of us had expected. She was a Clinical Research Associate (clinical drug trials monitor) with the opportunity to travel to support testing and approval of new pharmaceutical drugs. I had recently changed from engineering management to product management and worked mostly with utility companies in the electrical sector.

Actually, a major factor in the decision to accept the new position was to position myself for a general manager (GM) role and transition Rebecca to a *non-working* role. For about a year, I had actually been trying to convince her to shift to part time but had experienced a significant lack of success. Becca loved her job and she was good at it.

One day earlier, Becca had been working from her hospital room and I was working at home. We had both finished around the same time and she had told me not to come in because she was tired and planned to catch up on some sleep. This was a bit unusual but it would be good for her to rest. Besides, she would then be ready for our big New Year's Eve celebration, which would most likely consist of tapioca pudding and a movie on the laptop that we would pause every twenty-five minutes when the nurse came in.

Scanning the DVR recordings, it was clear we were way behind on our shows, and that I had recorded a large collection of movies that I had little interest in watching. Unfortunately, a day of moderately interesting movies and some minor cleaning was not in the cards. My phone rang and I saw it was Rebecca calling.

To my surprise, it was not Rebecca—it was the doctor. I knew immediately that something was wrong because the doctors never called me. Rebecca knew her condition inside and out, knew her medical history, and knew her treatment plans and medications. I couldn't add anything of value. The only reason for the doctor to call me was because Rebecca could not.

Becca had a very bad night. The oxygen saturation levels (sats) in her blood had declined overnight, despite increasing the level of her supplemental oxygen. This meant that her lung function had diminished significantly. To counter this, they had placed her on BiPAP and brought her to the MICU. I did not know what those unusual words meant, but I knew that things were bad. When the doctor is clearly uncomfortable giving you news, it is bad news. He asked if I was coming in and I said I was. There was something to his tone that suggested that this could be the last time I would see Rebecca. It hit me right in the chest. There was nothing at all 'routine' about this tune-up.

I went upstairs to get dressed. I came downstairs without my pants. I went back upstairs to find a different shirt. I came back down to look for my backpack. After what seemed like an eternity (but was probably closer to five minutes) I was marginally closer to being ready to leave. This was when I made myself stop. In that moment I realized that all I had to do was show up. I did not have to bring a bunch of supplies. I did not need to perform any kind of surgery. In fact, I did not need to know what to do. This was the first of many major lessons I learned as this nightmare began:

Lesson 1: Show up.

CHAPTER 1

Homework for Dating

Rebecca and I had learned many lessons prior to this point as well. We had been together for almost seventeen years and, like any relationship, there was a learning curve. We had met at the University of Connecticut in January of 1998. Rebecca told me early on in our relationship that she had CF and asked me if I knew what it was. I told her of course I did…but…perhaps I didn't remember all of the specific details so it would be fine if she wanted to refresh my memory. Okay, technically, I had no idea what the disease entailed but I had heard of it. Probably. I was certain that she could not see through my façade.

She saw fit to provide me with an eight-page technical article on the disease. This is the challenge with dating a cytogenetics major. I had not previously needed to do homework to date somebody, but she was worth it so I gave it a read. Being an experienced engineering student, I knew how to portray understanding and when I discussed the article with her, I was sure to mention the CFTR gene and its effect on protein production. She was quite impressed.

I learned that cystic fibrosis is a genetic disease caused by the body's inability to correctly produce a certain protein. This protein, called the Cystic Fibrosis Transmembrane Conductance Regulator

(CFTR), is responsible for transporting sodium chloride across cell membranes. As a result, the mucus that the body produces is thicker in someone with CF and causes damage to several organs.

The pancreas for example, often does not release digestive enzymes with food so people with CF usually need to take these enzymes in pill form with their meals and snacks. Even with that support, their bodies often do not absorb enough nutrients from their food and they can be smaller and undernourished. In some cases, like Rebecca's, they can develop CF-related diabetes (CFRD) as the pancreas can no longer secrete sufficient insulin to counter their carbohydrate intake. She developed this at sixteen years old and had to manage it closely every day.

The mucus in the lungs is also thicker and more difficult to clear (cough out) resulting in an ever-present cough and frequent lung infections. This is the driving factor behind many of the hospitalizations and the need for IV antibiotics. I always felt like I could pick her out of a lineup blindfolded because I knew the sound of her cough so well. It had a base that kicked in about a half second after it started followed by a long exhale.

The sinuses are also impacted, often developing polyps and infection. For Rebecca, this has led to severe headaches and over a dozen painful sinus surgeries. As a result, she lost her sense of smell, requiring me to smell all of her leftovers (including nasty food that I do not like) to inform her if they are still good. This is a burden that I have to shoulder alone.

The life expectancy for someone with this disease has increased significantly over her lifetime, in a large part due to the efforts of the Cystic Fibrosis Foundation (CFF). When Rebecca was born, she wasn't expected to survive until high school. Advances in care and development of new treatments and antibiotics have continued to prolong the life expectancy of people with CF. By the time we met, her life expectancy was around thirty.

To inherit cystic fibrosis, you must receive a mutated CFTR gene from each parent (the condition is recessive). Parents of someone with cystic fibrosis may not have CF themselves, but each carry at least one copy of the faulty gene. There are different severities along with various mutations of the disease. Rebecca has two copies of the most common mutation, Delta F508.

Becca was able to tell me her specific mutation because she had it tested. She had a strong interest in human biology driven by her own illness. She majored in cytogenetics and molecular biology, graduated Magna Cum Laude and was one of thirty University Scholars at the University of Connecticut (UConn). In other words, she was wicked smart, which explains why she wanted to date me.

We were halfway through our junior year when we met and had great chemistry from the start. We attended UConn and lived in a group of dorms affectionately called The Jungle. We met at a floor party on the day my niece Gabrielle was born. Apparently, Becca liked the fact that I was quite excited about this and bragging about my niece at the party.

This particular night, my friend Rui was "working on" Becca's friend, Melissa, and his efforts resulted in a group of girls partying on our floor. Contrary to logic, our studly group of friends did not often have large groups of girls on the floor.

During that first night, Becca and I learned that we had matching 1990 Chevy Luminas (surprisingly the least stolen car in America), she learned that I was a bouncer at the Civic Pub (the coolest bar on campus), and I learned that she liked to drink White Russians and had CF.

Over the next weeks, we met for coffee, had a few dates, and came to know each other's friends better. My favorite times were the meals. I distinctly remember going to brunch early on and thinking she would be surprised by the amount of food I had taken. I had two overloaded plates and four drinks (small glasses). But when we returned to our table, she had just as much food as I did! I looked at this girl who was 105 pounds (literally half my weight) and remember thinking, *Who is she trying to impress?*

I knew there was no way she could eat that much food and as I finished my first plate, she was only halfway through hers. She was just cutting tiny pieces, chatting, taking her time. I could not tell if she was slowing down, but it seemed like it. By the time I finished my second plate, she was finishing her first. So then I just sat there watching her chip away at it one little tiny piece at a time, just cutting, biting, and talking. When she was halfway done with her second plate, I was thoroughly impressed and began to wonder if she could actually finish it all. She just kept going! Before I knew it, she was sopping up the last remnant of syrup with her last piece of pancake, and it was done. Simply amazing.

Back in her room, I was surprised to find she had Slim Fast shakes. I learned that she used to drink them with meals for extra calories. She also had high-calorie Scandishakes that she would mix up with whole milk or cream. She gave some to our friend Big John when he broke his jaw during intramural softball and had it wired shut.

She began sitting at our table and my other friends got to know her. One morning, she came to the table with one plate of breakfast foods and a second filled exclusively with bacon. My friend, Norm, looked at it and asked so the rest of our group could hear, "Is that a full plate of bacon!?"

To which Bec replied without pause, "Shut up, Norm!"

"Hold on, that plate is piled with only bacon! You must really LOVE bacon." Norm said as he poked at her some more.

"You shut up, Norm. So…I like bacon."

"You must like it a lot."

"I do, and I'm going to eat all of it." And she did!

Yes, Becca fit into our group pretty well. Actually, that exchange became a running joke between her and Norm who always offered to make bacon for her when the opportunity arose.

It was greatly entertaining to be with a girl who was not sensitive when it came to food or her weight. Her strong love for Ben and Jerry's New York Superfudge Chunk inspired my first nickname for her—Superchunk. Though she did not like it in the traditional sense, it did not seem to bother her. To me, she was this little superhero who could eat whatever she wanted, was stronger than she looked, and was smart and spunky to boot. We just clicked.

The fact that we got along so well made me worry that she was the one. Early on, I had to make the call whether or not I should go through with a relationship that if successful, could end in heartbreak too soon. Thirty years old seemed like a long time away from twenty…but not long enough. I imagined dealing with the pain of loss and becoming a middle aged widower having to start my life over. That seemed scary and tragic. At the time, I thought early thirties was middle aged…but regardless, it was a very hard decision for me.

Was I assuming too much? Maybe it would not last that long. However, after a few short months, we were spending all of our free time together and not dating other people. I imagined breaking up and feeling like she was the one who got away. That was the point when I figured out the first of many lessons. With a lot of introspection, I decided that a more serious relationship was worth the risk. I did not want to be plagued with regret. I had figured out what I wanted.

Lesson 2: Sometimes you have to trust your instincts, take a risk, and not focus on the worst that could happen.

Becca had previously expressed that she was not interested in a long-term relationship, but being an expert on women, I understood that she was sure to change her mind. I had come to the conclusion that we should move forward. I knew she was quite smart, so I felt that, logically, she would come to the same conclusion. Having sorted this all out, I had the conversation.

Unbelievable as it was, she turned me down. She had just come out of two back-to-back long-term relationships and would be leaving for Virginia at the end of the year. This would be a six-month clinical

where she would work in a laboratory for some relevant real world experience. She was determined to not have the ties and complexities of a relationship when she left, so we continued to date, keeping the status quo.

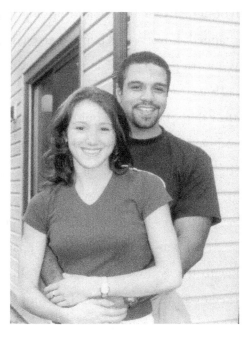

As the spring semester came to a close, I knew that I did not want to commute ninety minutes up to Storrs if we were not serious. I could meet someone local, save gas, and take advantage of the fact that my license would soon tell the world I was twenty-one. So on spring weekend, instead of heading to a kill-a-keg party together like we had planned, I went there with my friends and gave her a call from the party. It wasn't *that* far off campus and she could just meet me. She was…displeased. She did not come out that night and that was fine with me. The plan was in motion.

It was an easy way to start the breakup process. I decided that I was not going to drive up from Brookfield every weekend, so we might as well end it when the semester ended. I would be a little less agreeable, she would get annoyed with me, and then I could break it off nice and clean. It was a flawless plan.

Well, it was a nearly flawless plan. The next day, I felt guilty so I bought her a flower and apologized to her. My intentions had not changed, however. When we arrived at my place, I started "The Talk." We were going to be living apart during the summer. We would both be busy with work and friends. She was leaving for a clinical shortly after that. Then we would be living at a distance for over six months and we had not even dated that long. It was all coming out so well until she said, "OK. Let's do it."

"Uhh…let's do what?"

"Let's be exclusive. Let's agree not to date anyone else."

I was confused and unprepared because I had not planned for her to throw a curveball halfway through my well-rehearsed, brilliantly executed breakup speech. I had intended to let her down nice and easy (and maybe stay in touch for when she returned from clinical). Needless to say, my nearly flawless plan failed. Or I suppose you could say that my original plan succeeded. Yes, let's go with that.

Part of what I liked about her was her attitude. She had dealt with so many obstacles in her life yet she was unfazed. Once she left for college, she was on her own and self-sufficient (and had been since she was eighteen). She worked to pay her bills, earned scholarships with her academic performance, and still found time to hang out and enjoy life. She would get her college degree even though the math suggested that she would not live long enough to pay it back. She was determined to achieve her goals.

As in any relationship, the longer we were together, the more I learned about her motivations and who she was. For most of her life through college, Becca had stayed relatively healthy. She dealt with mealtime pills (digestive enzymes), insulin injections, breathing treatments, and coughing fits, but she managed to live an active life. She was incredibly motivated and focused on her academics. This was even more impressive after hearing her story.

Rebecca was born in Milford, Massachusetts, in 1977 to her mother Brenda, who was sixteen years old. Becca's father Scott was only three years older. In her first months, Rebecca was diagnosed with "failure to thrive." She almost died and was diagnosed with cystic fibrosis at six months old. At ten months old she weighed 11 pounds and was 24 inches tall (the size of an average two- or three-month-old). At less than a year old, she had experienced pneumonia, a pneumothorax (collapsed lung), and sepsis (organ injury from infection).

By two years old, her parents had divorced and she moved to Florida with her mom. It was there where her mom married Pete and her sister Jessica was born. Becca grew very close to him and he treated her like his own daughter. She always reflected on this time of her life with affection—except for the heat and sweating. Florida is damn hot.

She described herself as precocious and explained that she would always carry a purse around filled with "proper things." She would make her sister play school and office and was convinced that she was the reason why her sister hated school.

When Becca was seven, Brenda and Pete divorced, which was tough on her. Fortunately, visitations with Pete continued for both her and her sister which helped to ease the transition and provide some stability. She had grown extremely close to him and thought of him like a dad (rather than as a stepdad).

At ten, Rebecca was given the choice to stay with her mother in Florida or move in with her biological father Scott and Viola, her stepmother, in Maine. She chose Maine, partly because the situation was more stable. She remained there through high school. During the summers, she would often visit her mother, who had remarried and moved to Idaho.

Living in Maine was a major change from Florida. Her father and Vi were very religious and often strict. Scott was a quiet man who had learned the farrier trade (shoeing horses). This is tough work in the cold winters and he often put in many hours. Vi stayed home and was very involved with Becca's upbringing.

Becca was a good kid but often butted heads with Vi. She had come from a much less rigid environment and now she was not allowed to listen to her favorite Kenny Rogers and Heart cassettes—only Christian music. She had many chores maintaining the house along with taking care of the horses. In school she managed to maintain all As and, despite her lung disease, excelled on the cross country team.

From a young age, Becca developed a strong focus and the character that would shape her into the woman she became. In addition to all of her medical issues, Becca had a speech impediment. She had worked to overcome her stutter since childhood but still had good days and bad. Then at sixteen, she was diagnosed with cystic fibrosis related diabetes (CFRD). She became insulin dependent. She now had another daily challenge to face.

She struggled with the fact that she did not have the same social freedoms that other kids her age enjoyed. At one point, Vi told her she could not attend her senior prom with her boyfriend. She was relieved when her father stepped in and allowed it.

When describing her upbringing, Rebecca was always sure to mention that the stability of her home in Maine was good for her. She never regretted taking the steady route because she knew it was what she needed most at that time.

While Bec was in high school, her mother had two more children, Jordan and Hannah. Rebecca was thrilled at the idea of a little brother and another little sister. Though Brenda divorced again a few years later, Bec made sure to call them and send gifts on every birthday. She had a sense of responsibility that was impressive. By the time of her high school graduation, Becca was more mature than most others her age. She was determined to pay her way through college, and was completely independent once she arrived at the University of Connecticut. She had received several scholarships and student loans. She also got a part-time work-study job during the semester and worked full time over the summers. She was taking care of herself at eighteen years old while taking a tough course load and excelling. She was a force to be reckoned with.

At the same time, Brenda struggled through several failed relationships, turbulence at home, and the subsequent loss of custody of Jordan and Hannah. This created a challenging environment for

Rebecca's teenaged sister Jessica. After hearing some concerning stories from Jessica about their living situation, Rebecca did not want to cross her mother, but felt she needed to do something to watch out for her sister. She knew that Jessica should not stay in that environment and required something more safe and stable.

Though they had lived apart for several years, Rebecca adored her sister. They were different in many ways because Jessica was relaxed and more of a free spirit while Bec was very goal-oriented and focused. They were like a mini female Odd Couple.

Knowing that it would risk her relationship with her mother, she told her stepdad Pete about the situation. He immediately stepped up and took Jessica in to live with him in St. Louis. It took a lot of courage for Becca to stand up for Jessica and to involve her dad, but she saw it as black and white. Even though she was young and barely on her own, she was resolute and knew what she had to do. As a repercussion, her mother did not talk to her for about a year. Becca dealt with this in her typical, realistic fashion. She missed her interaction with Brenda, but knew that her actions were necessary. It was soon after that I met Rebecca. We did not talk about it much since Bec knew she had done nothing wrong and was so focused on what she needed to do at college. Meanwhile, she continued her efforts to stay in touch with Jordan and Hannah and was even able to plan occasional visits with them. I remember learning her story and being surprised that she was so well grounded.

Just before our one year anniversary, she left for her clinical in Virginia. It seemed unfair that she needed to pay full tuition (even though she was not taking traditional classes), work a forty-hour-per-week clinical for no pay, and then get a part-time job on top of that to cover room and board. She managed it by pushing herself past her limit. Up to that point, I knew her signature cough but I had not really seen her sick. Her body was tired from working so many hours while getting too little sleep. As the spring arrived, I listened over the phone while she coughed so much more and had almost no voice. I tried to convince her to work less but as I would come to learn over the years, I am less convincing than I give myself credit for.

Pushing past limits makes for great inspirational posters, but loses its luster when your girlfriend ends up in the hospital with pneumonia 400 miles away. I traveled down to visit her in the hospital and was surprised to see how truly sick she had become. I remember walking toward her room and seeing an incredibly skinny arm reach up toward a nurse. As I got closer, I realized it was Becca. She was petite to begin with, but the weight loss from pneumonia made a significant impact on how she looked. I realized that I could not leave her there. She would work out the details of the final weeks of her clinical with UConn and the institution, but her health was first and foremost.

She was discharged with home IVs and I asked my parents if she could come and stay with us for the last weeks of the summer. They had only met Rebecca a few times at that point but they were happy to help. They knew her story, clicked with her personality, and had a great deal of respect for her. As soon as she was healthy enough, I loaded up our two Chevy Luminas (mine being the Eurosport edition) with all of her things. We set up Bec with her IV antibiotics and I duct taped her insulin pen to the AC vent (which I later learned was unnecessary) and we started the drive back to my parents' house in Danbury.

Typical expectations would be that a twenty-one-year-old college student renting a pre-furnished apartment would not have a lot of things. This was not the case. Rebecca had THINGS. She loved to shop and get discounts and introduced me to the term "retail therapy." Needless to say, the packing of our Luminas was an amazing engineering feat, only possibly rivaled by Edison or Da Vinci. We could even see out of the car windows!

That whole experience drove the point home that getting enough rest was essential to her staying healthy. Over the years, I would see it occur again and again. Her CF exacerbations would often be preceded by a period of insufficient sleep and too much stress.

It was back at my family's house in Danbury that Rebecca saw her mother for the first time in several years. They had never really settled what had happened, and they had just started talking again. She did not have much money, so my parents said she could stay with us as well.

A peek into Becca's closet triggered a lecture from Brenda who told her that she was too materialistic and should spend less on her clothes. She compared Bec's budget to her own, which she suggested was better managed. By this time, Becca had been paying for both her college tuition and living expenses for three years with very little financial help from anyone. Her father Scott helped as much as he could with tuition, but for the most part Becca managed on her own.

Brenda was not completely wrong, Rebecca had a few too many sundresses from T.J. Maxx, but it came across as a parent scolding a reckless teenager. Rebecca was an adult who had handled everything life threw at her, and this lady who had not played a prominent role for eleven years was preaching at her.

I prepared myself for the intense Becca response that I had come to know, but it never came. If anyone else had done that she would have told them where they could stick it. Nobody was helping her with her bills and she was clearly capable of managing them. She did not come back with the bold confidence that I had come to expect, she only acknowledged that Brenda was probably right.

Perhaps it was because she had seen her mother so infrequently since she was ten, maybe it was the year of Brenda's silence, but it seemed that Becca was willing to deal with it to maintain the relationship. Perhaps I was an engineering student and Psych 101 did not give me a full enough arsenal to psychoanalyze their relationship over one long weekend. Ultimately, it was their relationship and I was not about to pry.

In any case, we would only see Brenda one more time before we graduated. She had just gotten married again, and was passing through with her new husband. I cannot remember his name; just that they seemed like a poor match on so many levels. It was clear to me that Brenda was very driven by emotion and impulse. I think this had been good for Rebecca years earlier, when Brenda kept pushing until the doctors diagnosed what was wrong. I did not need to understand Brenda to know that without her, Becca would not be here. Beyond that, she was fun to hang out and have some drinks with. She was quite a character and it was nice to feel that I could talk freely and did not have to watch what I said. We got along well. Interestingly, her actions drew a sharp contrast with those of Rebecca's. I found it impressive that Rebecca turned out as grounded as she did in the face of such an unusual personality.

Graduation came faster than we could imagine. More time together had meant more time to see how this progressive disease worked. Fortunately, it worked slowly during that time. I saw her through several sinus surgeries, but that was typically less than once per year. It was still tough to hear her coughing fits but I became more used to it with time. Early on, she would comment, "I'm dying." I knew she meant nothing by it, but her mortality was so much on my mind that the comment was piercing. My mind would instantly flash forward to this perceived future loss. This feeling gradually decreased with time as her situation became part of the norm for us.

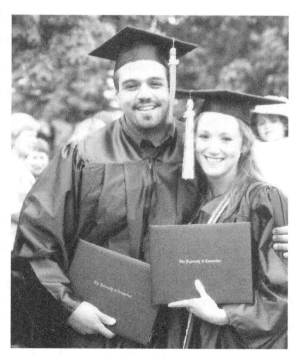

CHAPTER 2

Getting Serious

As with any relationship, it is natural to get into arguments or have disagreements over each person's roles and responsibilities. In that respect, our relationship was no different. We both had very strong opinions but we also did a good job in finding common ground. "Pick your battles" became our unofficial mantra in this area. I felt that in many ways, Rebecca's illness gave me perspective through these times, helping me to keep my eye on the bigger picture. However, there was still a learning curve.

Initially, empathy for someone you care about makes you want to give them everything they want. The logic is that time is precious and there is no need to waste it arguing about the little things. In the end, it is all little things. As bad as it sounds, I would often try view it from the perspective of myself looking back after she was gone. Would this have mattered? Was it worth arguing about the fact that she wanted to try some new, expensive wine with dinner? It was better to just agree with her and let it go.

That logic would work for a little while, then the feelings of resentment would kick in. When I reasoned that it was not worth an argument, I was also reasoning that it was not worth arguing for my opinion. During times that I took that stance out of guilt or to avoid regret, frustration would build. That feeling could continue for only so long before I found myself re-starting an argument on the subject because I needed to have my side understood. The feeling that I had to withhold my words because she was a delicate flower did not hold water. She did not present herself that way nor did she argue that way. In fact, she prided herself on being tough, as do so many people with CF. She was half of a partnership but I was the other half.

Lesson 3: Pick your battles but argue for the things that matter to you; it is better than holding a grudge.

The perspective that CF brought was that there was little time. We needed to approach each other with respect for the other's perspective. Maybe we would never see eye-to-eye but if we could develop a running rule, we would be fine. For example, we could try to find new, good wines at the store but when we were out for dinner, we would just find a good pairing. That way it doesn't have to ruin the next date night.

There is a possibility that these were not groundbreaking relationship developments, but it worked because we worked on it. Ultimately, I wanted to look back at our time together and feel I had given it my best shot and had no major regrets. This may be a morbid way to look at a relationship but whenever I did, I could use reason to guide me toward the best path. It seemed to work for me.

When it came to her health, the most immediate issue was

often her blood sugar. Bec put a lot of effort into managing this and she would try to keep her blood sugars in a tight range—80 to 120 mg/dl. She was also very small with little body fat. As I would later learn, this would contribute to her being a brittle diabetic, which meant that her blood sugar could change quickly. Seemingly minor mistakes could have fast and severe effects. She carried a glucometer to test her blood sugar and over the years, used needles, an insulin pen, and finally an insulin pump to manage her injections. Every three months, she would have a blood test called hemoglobin A1c that would indicate how well her blood sugar was controlled.

Low blood sugar was risky and could cause someone to slip into a coma with the worst case being death. If her blood sugar fell too low (hypoglycemia), she would get disoriented or find it hard to concentrate. She would typically know if it was going low but not every time. This was a scary reality and became scarier when considering that it could happen when she was driving. I could sometimes tell it was low when we were talking. If she had a tough time trying to understand a simple concept, we would stop and test.

Going high meant that she was experiencing hyperglycemia (not marijuana). It did not lead to the same immediate concern as a low blood sugar but over time, it could lead to neuropathy (nerve damage) or even amputation of the extremities. Not taking enough insulin with meals was the major cause, but sickness and certain medications—like prednisone or other steroids—would also drive her blood sugar high. High levels made it difficult to gain weight as well. She could usually tell if her blood sugar was high when she had extreme thirst that she could not seem to quench. Though she would do her best to manage it, sometimes she would get focused on work and forget to eat or occasionally eat and forget to take insulin. Forgetting insulin is one thing but I *never* understood how she could forget to eat. I often remembered to eat hours before I even required food.

When she would go low, she would get to go through the cabinet and find the junkiest, most sugary deliciousness and eat it in front of me. In a show of support, I would also eat whatever junky delight she would discover. Since I attempted to eat healthy most of the time, this was clearly a selfless act on my part.

She had one instance of low blood sugar when I was driving. She argued she would just have some candy when we got home in ten minutes. I stopped anyway and dropped her at the door of the grocery store to quickly grab some snacks while I parked. In my rearview mirror, I could see her walking with an odd limp. I hopped out of the jeep and raced into the store to find her sitting on a bench at the entrance. She had forgotten why she was there. I bought some skittles and as she ate them she slowly came back to reality. I imagined what could have happened if she was driving and decided to go home. She could be in an accident somewhere and even if it was just a fender bender, her blood sugar would just continue to drop. We needed a better plan.

The next day, we went to Costco and bought a case of skittles. We put them everywhere: her pocketbook, night stand, both of our cars. We always had skittles with us and we would bring them out at the slightest sign of a low blood sugar. She came to hate skittles. We eventually switched to juice boxes, but from then on we had a plan.

With college behind us and over three years as a couple, there was a new challenge on the horizon: marriage. I still held one main concern as I made this decision. I knew that with CF, there was a strong chance that she would not be able to have children. I had always wanted kids. Of course if we had problems, there was always in vitro fertilization (IVF). Additionally, if we had kids and she passed away when they were young, I knew it would be tough on them and I would be left alone to raise them. In the end, I knew I had no guarantees that this would not be the case even with somebody else. The only difference was that here I knew the odds. Knowing that we could not plan for everything, we would just have to figure that out when the time came. She was worth it to me, so it was just a matter of when to pop the question.

We both had our plans as far as the timing. I was going to give it a little time and enjoy going out with my friends since we had just graduated. Rebecca had moved into a nice place up in Branford with a roommate, buying me plenty of time to make my decision. When I was ready, I would find the right moment and ask. It was a solid plan.

Rebecca's plan was similar but had several more specifics. She decided that she wanted a fall wedding. She also determined that she needed eighteen months to plan appropriately, and then presented me with a date by which time I should propose. She had also made it clear that she wanted a princess cut diamond with two smaller stones on the side and a platinum ring. The carat weight was not important, but ideally, it would look "antique-ish." She said the rest was up to me, though it did not seem like there was much else. She provided me with the specifications frequently and would even quiz me to ensure I remembered the details. Her ring size, however, was provided only once. As the time came closer for me to propose I could not ruin the surprise and ask.

Her proposal target date came and went. When her birthday arrived in June, I thought a mountain bike would be the perfect gift. We could spend time together riding on the trails and it would be a great workout. Surprisingly, she was not as excited about my gift as I had expected. Perhaps it was because she was expecting something else.

Not long afterward, I was ready to buy a ring. The challenge was that I did not know her ring size and could not ask her without arousing suspicion. Like a good engineer, I snuck into her jewelry box with my digital calipers and measured the inside diameters of several of her rings, averaged them together, calculated the circumference, then used an online chart to determine the size. The result did not feel right because the standard deviation was too large and the average was quite far from what I had anticipated. It turned out that they were rings worn on all different fingers. So in the end, I guessed. I went to New Jersey with my brother-in-law Michael, to where he had purchased my sister's ring. I found the perfect one.

I decided to propose at a party she was hosting with her work friends one Friday night. I had the ring shipped to my sister Rachel's house and had to pick it up before arriving. She had given me a rose from her garden, some champagne, and two flutes for the big moment.

It was going to be a big night with a private proposal and a party afterward to make it public. It was another perfect plan.

Traveling on I-95 on Friday at rush hour was not exactly ideal and I showed up late to an annoyed girlfriend. As I got dressed, she came into her room and started cleaning up after me. She grabbed my shirt and went to put it in my duffel bag. The ring, rose, and all of the goodies were on the top of the bag and she was seconds away from ruining her surprise. As she reached for the zipper, I had to act quickly. I stopped her with, "Why do you always have to clean up? I'll pick up my own stuff, just leave me alone and let me get ready!"

Success and failure. She tossed my shirt down with a, "Fine!" and stomped out. Good job, me.

The night went on and I knew the time was not right. Between getting a subtle sense of the mood and feel of the event coupled with the fact that she got super drunk, I brilliantly determined that it would be best to delay the proposal and focus on catching up to her buzz level.

The next morning while she was cleaning downstairs, I laid out a rose on the bed and set the champagne and flutes on her night stand. At this point, the champagne was just for show because we were both way too hungover to partake. I called her up and she ignored me, still unhappy about my lateness and attitude the night before.

I asked her roommate to call her and she came right up. She stopped in the doorway, squinting at the bed in disbelief. I pulled her into the room and closed the door. I intended to get down on one knee, but she was so stunned that she was shaky on her feet and looked like she might tip over. As I stood there holding her up, I asked her to marry me, she just cried. I knew that meant *yes* even though I did not get my answer for a minute or two.

The next year flew by. Even though Rebecca did not have eighteen months to plan the wedding, it was a success. The day came and Rebecca looked beautiful. My best man Norm gave an amazing wedding speech that nobody could forget. The slideshow I put together was a hit. Not a detail was missed and everybody was there. Rebecca danced with her dad and her stepdad. I danced with my mom and had a dance off with my dad. It was perfect.

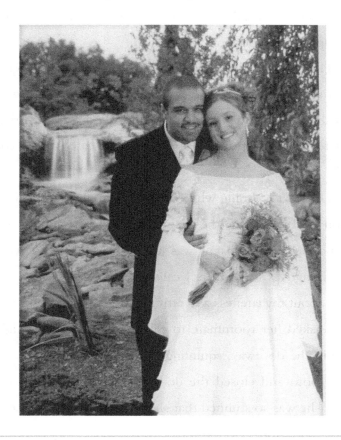

CHAPTER 3

False-Starting a Family

We had an amazing honeymoon in Aruba, but not long after we returned, it was announced that the Remington Shaver plant in Bridgeport, Connecticut, where I worked, was being shut down. This meant I would either have to accept a corporate relocation to Wisconsin, or join my recently laid off wife on the couch. We opted for the move.

Becca found a job quickly. She had decided that lab work was not for her and set her sights on becoming a clinical drug trials monitor. She was able to get an entry level position at a company in Madison and after a year and a half, she was offered the position she had wanted.

The University of Wisconsin (UW) hospital provided great CF care and Rebecca was a compliant patient. She did all of her breathing treatments, managed her blood sugar, paid close attention to sinus issues, took her digestive enzymes, while at the same time working full time. It was around this time when she started with her tune-ups. UW focused on prevention and when she would start to feel sick, they would act quickly to put her on IV antibiotics.

At the time, this would happen about once per year. She would go in the hospital for about two weeks and come out much healthier. The only problem was that it is tough to get good rest in the hospital because the nurses come in the room around the clock for a variety of reasons. She would occasionally do these IVs at home. This was much more work on our end (mostly Rebecca's end) depending on the timing of her meds. She would often have to wake up in the middle of the night to infuse a dose. The benefit was that she was in the comfort of her own home.

My biggest complaint was the fact that she could not slow down. She was supposed to be home resting and she would be puttering around the kitchen, cleaning her office, checking emails, basically trying to check things off of her to-do list. I found myself chasing her back to bed ALL the time. She recovered the quickest when she was getting her sleep and not overexerting herself, but she had a busy mind.

During these tune-ups, they would typically place something called a Peripherally Inserted Central Catheter, or a PICC line. This is a long catheter placed intravenously that allows for infusions for a prolonged period of time. It would be placed in her arm and the catheter, which was about two feet long, would extend to just over her heart.

Toward the end of one tune-up, Becca had to leave for a business trip the morning after her last infusion. She was done with her regimen of antibiotics and ready to get the PICC line out. If she kept it, she would have to flush it daily with saline and heparin (anti-clotting medication). She decided that this was too much of a hassle and that we could pull it out ourselves.

I am not sure where she got this idea but she proposed it to me with a great deal of confidence. "You just have to put pressure on the insertion point and pull it out at a slow consistent rate," she told me. It took some convincing but I finally agreed to help her with it. She sat on the toilet and I positioned myself in front of her. First I removed the dressing and clipped the stitches holding the end in place. Becca was such a seasoned patient and do-it-yourselfer that she sat there with all of the confidence in the world. I put pressure on the site then started to slowly pull. Then things went bad.

When a little of her warm blood dripped onto her leg, she started to get light headed. She tipped forward toward me with her eyes still open, beginning a slow moaning exhale. I had one hand holding gauze at the insertion, and the other hand pulling the PICC out (at a slow steady pace) so I was forced to catch her between my neck and shoulder. I still had to keep pulling but now in this new position, I loosened my grip on the gauze and more blood started flowing out. Had *The Walking Dead* begun to air, I would have been more cautious about exposing my neck to her, but her moans were unnerving regardless. I finally got the rest of the line out and increased pressure on the site. I waited and watched while she slowly stopped moaning and started blinking a little more. As she was looking at me I could see her slowly reappear behind her eyes. She was confused, wondering what had happened. There was blood in her lap and all over the toilet. Her PICC line was on the floor as I knelt in front of her in our bathroom waiting for her to be alert enough to tell her, "NEVER

AGAIN! I WILL NEVER DO THAT AGAIN!!! EVER."

"That was weird." she told me.

"WEIRD?! That was weird!?! Do you know what happened? I will never, ever, ever do that again. That was awful!"

"I've turned into a weenie." She told me.

"You've missed my point entirely. If the apocalypse comes and you have a PICC line, we will roam the earth looking for saline, heparin, and alcohol pads because I am never pulling one of these again." I was stuck in a precarious situation with nobody else around performing a pseudo-medical procedure that SHE had talked me into...and she was reflecting on how she used to be tougher!?!

From that point forward, I stuck to my no PICC line removal stance and have never compromised. Some days when I would think of it, often when she got a new PICC placed, I would proactively remind her of my uncompromising position and that she would never convince me to remove it. She would roll her eyes at me unfazed by my bold stance. I would later learn that she had experienced a panic attack. This info would do me no good but at least I had an explanation.

It was not long after we moved to Wisconsin that we decided to start a family. Rebecca was the first to say she wanted a baby, though she worried about her fertility as a result of CF. She figured the sooner the better while she was still healthy enough. Our main concern was her well-being. Would she be healthy enough to carry a baby and if so, would the pregnancy cause any negative long-term ramifications?

My other concern was her life expectancy. I had to be ready to take on full responsibility of this child at any time. We were twenty-six and the average life expectancy for someone with CF was in the early to mid-thirties. I needed to determine why I wanted a child. It could not be about appeasing Rebecca because I would ultimately be a single father with all of this responsibility on my shoulders.

I wondered if it was fair to bring a child into the world knowing that its mother might not be around to see it off to school. I reasoned that life is a blessing and that we would do our best for this child. I remembered that they thought Becca would not make it to high school and here we were in our mid-twenties. I also remembered my reasoning from when I decided to get together with Rebecca. It is impossible to predict the future so I did not want that to paralyze myself in the present. Anyone can get hit by a car tomorrow but that should not stop you from living today. We had heard that there were people with CF who were in their fifties and some who had children. We needed to live our lives. I was ready.

We went to her CF doctor and discussed this with him. He told us that there was not any major risk to Rebecca at the time. She was healthy, and as long as she continued to be compliant, he would expect her to do well. He commented on how much help she would need from me which was something I had expected and would gladly provide. He eased our fears about the process but stressed that she would need to let others help her. She was accepting of this and we even talked about the potential of asking her mother to stay with us for a few months after the birth.

We were aware that many women with CF had trouble getting pregnant but we were going to give it our best shot. Rebecca and I were excited about the possibility of a child. As always, she did her research—lots and lots of research. She took temperature measurements to know when she was ovulating, she took prenatal vitamins, went to an acupuncturist...whatever we could do to make this happen, we were going to try. My job was pretty simple but being a good husband, I was willing to "help" when called upon. In fact I had a standing offer of "help."

At the same time, her mom and sister were trying to convince her not to do it. Despite what the doctor said, they worried that this was going to weaken her and shorten her life. Brenda told her it was selfish of me to push her toward this and Jessica worried she would not accept anyone else's help. Technically, it was Rebecca pulling me toward this but I suppose the in-law is always going to be the bad guy.

After trying for several months, we recognized that we would need the support of a fertility doctor. The issue appeared to be CF related. We decided to start with a process called intrauterine insemination (IUI). The process itself was simple but waiting two weeks to see of it had worked was draining. They told us that if it did not work by the third try, we would need to try something else.

Then on the first try, it worked! We were so thrilled at the possibility of having a baby. It all seemed so surreal. We started to really imagine what it would be like and we were anxious for the first trimester to be over so we could start to tell people. Unfortunately, our celebration would be short-lived. We lost it soon after, and Rebecca was heartbroken. We tried to focus on the positive side: it had worked. If it worked so easily this time, we were bound to succeed eventually.

We went back for a second and third round but to our disappointment, nothing came of it. At this point the doctors told us that our best option was in vitro fertilization (IVF).

We went for two rounds of IVF with no results. We planned on doing a third round, but our insurance would no longer cover the procedure so we didn't go through with it. It felt like we were so close, but positive results were elusive. Time between procedures had stretched longer and longer because of the time it took to recover emotionally from each failure. We began to realize that we had two real options left—surrogacy or adoption.

I had considered adoption several times and struggled with a final decision. *Do I want children?* was not the right question. It was *WHY do I want children?* It took a lot of reflection, but I decided that I wanted children because I wanted a part of us to live on. I also wanted to always have a part of Rebecca with me. I admired those loving parents who chose adoption, but it did not line up with the reason why I wanted a child. Maybe one day those feelings would change, but at that point and in our situation, I did not want to adopt.

The other option was surrogacy. To our excitement Jessica agreed to be our surrogate. We still had some embryos in storage from the IVF sessions and once we were ready, we could pull the trigger. Jessica already had a son Cole, who was now a few years old. She was getting married and told us that she would want to wait until after she had a child with her husband. A few months later, she told us that she had changed her mind. It was tough news to take.

She had conflicting feelings as to the reasons for her decision which included the concern that Rebecca would wear herself out with a child. Rebecca knew that she needed a lot of support with this child but that was something that would have to be taken at her word. I also knew that she would do better as a stay-at-home mom rather than continuing to travel and work crazy hours, particularly because we could help her with a child. On the contrary, when she had to get a report filed by midnight then pack a suitcase for the next day, she was on her own.

Jessica also felt that I should be willing to adopt first. She changed her mind a few more times but ultimately she decided not to do it. This was an emotional roller coaster for the two of us as we switched back and forth from having a plan to not knowing what was next. Our friend Meg also offered and so did Rebecca's other sister Hannah. It was incredibly selfless for Jessica, Meg, and Hannah to offer to make one of the biggest sacrifices someone could make for someone else. But as time passed we questioned whether this was what we still wanted.

Rebecca had become so much more involved in a career that she loved and I started to worry about our chances of success with the procedure. A surrogate could cost tens of thousands of dollars and after paying for IVF medications, I was in no hurry to gamble on another "chance." Time passed and Rebecca had more frequent exacerbations and tune-ups. She had little energy outside of work, which consumed so much of her time. We spoke about it less and less as her health began to decline.

CHAPTER 4

The OC

When we moved to Oconomowoc (pronounced just like it's spelled), Wisconsin, Rebecca was averaging two tune-ups per year. She had increased gastrointestinal (GI) issues which resulted in stomach pain with many of her meals. Eating less, she struggled to maintain her weight.

At this time, I was in graduate school getting my MBA. I loved engineering but I had decided I ultimately wanted to be a general manager at a manufacturing company. My goal was to achieve this before I was forty. Between the two of us, we spent a lot of time working. The more we did, the easier it was to let the baby conversation shift to the back burner. We never made a final decision but time ultimately decided for us.

Rebecca loved her job monitoring clinical drug trials as a Clinical Research Associate and was able to work from home and travel almost every week. She monitored all phases of drug testing and ensured that sites administered the drugs appropriately and followed the protocol. She ensured that patients qualified and consented to the study, the regulatory paperwork was signed and in order, patients were protected, data was accurate, and the study site was prepared for any

FDA audits. With her type-A personality, the job was a great fit. She could organize stacks of papers and compare them with other stacks of papers. She had tons of files and drawers for her files. She had different color sticky notes and highlighters. This was perfect for her. I would jump out of the highest window I could find if I had the job but she absolutely loved it!

In the meantime, Brenda had recently remarried and her husband Rich got a job nearby. We offered to have them stay with us during this time, and they paid us a modest amount that was helpful right after the move. They typically travelled and stayed in a fifth-wheel trailer somewhere near the job site, but this was an opportunity for Rebecca and her mom to have some time together. We had an in-law suite downstairs, complete with a full second kitchen and there was plenty of space for us all. It went well. I got the chance get to know Rich better. He turned out to be a great guy. It was nice to have someone around to grab a beer with and to have a second set of hands around the house. They were only there for a few months which passed quickly.

It was not long before a medical evaluation revealed that she required a machine called a concentrator to provide supplemental oxygen (O_2) at night. Her O_2 levels would drop under 90 percent while she was sleeping and exercising, and she needed the oxygen to keep her sats up. This was a tough piece of news to take. It was nice to have the accompanying handicap parking, but it wasn't quite worth the tradeoff.

Soon afterward, she cultured Burkholderia cepacia (B. cepacia), a very bad strain of bacteria. We were able to knock it out with multiple rounds of aggressive antibiotics but we worried that it would affect her future chances of getting listed for a lung transplant. Though she struggled more and more every day, a transplant still seemed far off in the future. We focused on enjoying the present.

Our new house in Oconomowoc (the OC) was perfectly set up for my annual Big Barbeque (BBBQ). The finished basement had space for my pool table and a tile floor for spilling drinks. I splurged and bought a badminton set so I could show our guests what a true champion looked like on the court. Each year the event became larger as I invited new friends.

I was more social while Rebecca preferred nights at home on the couch. We found common ground, though it had less to do with our compromise skills and more to do with her frequent travel schedule. I could maintain an active social calendar when she was traveling and we would plan things together when she was not. I would periodically encourage her to go out with her friends for a change of pace and to get the shopping out of her system. We were really enjoying life in Oconomowoc, which is also known as the 5-O since there are five Os in Oconomowoc.

As her health continued to decline, she had a decreasing desire to leave the house outside of work. We would select a few events to attend and settled into a close group of friends with whom we would make plans. Together we went to Napa Valley and Key West and were always discussing and planning our next trip. It was made up of people I worked with: Stephanie, Meagan, Melanie, and Melanie's husband Mike...our awesome fire chief friend.

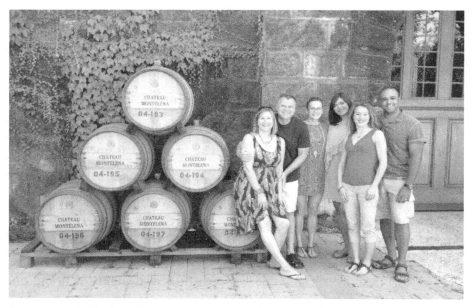

Left to right: Melanie, Mike, Meagan, Stephanie, Rebecca, Raymond

When Mike and Melanie told us they were attending a wine tasting event that was organized by the Cystic Fibrosis Foundation, Bec and I were game. It was there where we met Danelle, the director of the Wisconsin CFF chapter, who told me about the Milwaukee's Finest event.

Milwaukee's Finest was the CFF version of Person of the Year and it was all new territory for me. The event was in recognition of young professionals who volunteered in their community. We would learn more about CF and fundraise to support the CFF. I had previously led United Way efforts in my company and had often considered doing something with the CFF. I started fundraising and planning events and really enjoyed it. I had been sort of waiting for Rebecca to want to participate but when I started working on the

Finest campaign, I realized that she did not need to be involved. It related to her, but this could be my thing.

It was rewarding to do something for a great cause and organization. The CFF has driven much of the progress that has been made toward treating and curing the disease. They run their own labs, work with pharmaceutical companies, and have many programs that help the CF community. They use their funding efficiently and the people that work there truly care about curing this disease.

I organized a self-defense night with Salick's Karate, an innovative martial arts school that I was attending at the time in Delafield, Wisconsin. The sensei there volunteered to do it for free then he and all of the other instructors volunteered and donated as well. My sister Rachel and her family did a bake sale outside of their GNC store in Greenwich, Connecticut. My company donated a nice amount, which was matched by my buddies Norm and Alex who donated way more than I expected. I planned a bar event near Milwaukee and had a great turnout. Apparently, people like to drink booze and can be very generous after doing so! I was overwhelmed by support and surprised by my success. We had raised over $10,000 for the CFF and I won the distinction of being Milwaukee's finest. I had five minutes of solid fame when I was featured on the "Making Milwaukee Great" segment of our local news station.

It was a little bittersweet because as all of this was happening, Becca's condition was continuing to worsen. The next weekend, we vacationed in Newport with our friends, Dom and Steph, and she struggled just walking to the sights there. We had to walk at a pace so slow that it barely felt like we were moving. I considered calling a cab to go a half a mile but Becca refused. It was a scary sign of things to come.

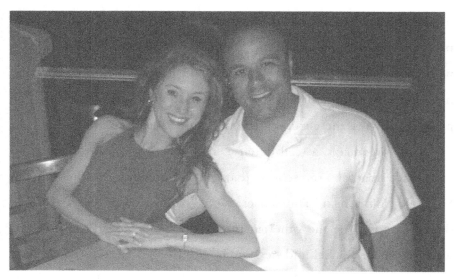

As the next year passed, Rebecca began to travel less due to her medical condition and I started to look for a new position. I was ready to leave the cold winters of Wisconsin behind, but she was wary. I had to negotiate relocation options with her, state by state. She did not want to live in any place too far south because she had to have all four seasons. This was understandable because she loved snow. When the winter hit, she would hope and pray for it. This way, she had something pretty to look at out the window before she walked down the stairs to her cozy office. This would usually happen a few hours after I woke up early to shovel the driveway and sidewalks then drove off to work.

Sometimes when it snowed at night, she would have me light the gas fireplace. Then, after I shoveled the walk around the house, the walk to the front door, and the driveway, she would poke her head out to remind me to salt for the cleaning people or shovel closer to the mailbox. When it was done she would be waiting to give me a nice warm hug. Even living in the Wisconsin winter wonderland that we enjoyed, I nevertheless developed some desire to move.

I received a few offers but ultimately accepted a position in the greater Cincinnati area. It was a good compromise—closer to my family in Connecticut, no farther from Jessica in St. Louis, a little warmer, and the hospital and associated CF clinic was good. More than that, though, I had found a position where I could grow into a General Manager role and this was a great opportunity. This had been my goal for over ten years and had motivated me to get my MBA. I was excited at the prospect of this happening before I was forty. Everyone needs an arbitrary goal.

Rebecca would not be working for much longer. We had estimated that it would be maybe another year or two before she would need to slow down and be ready for a lung transplant. A general manager role would allow me to provide the same lifestyle to which we had become accustomed, even after she stopped working. I figured I would have about two to three years under my belt at the new job before we needed to worry about the transplant.

Before the move we had a big vacation to Hawaii planned. It was booked for May of 2014. During Bec's packing (or over-packing) process, I was living in Cincinnati so I would avoid the usual chaos of her selections. I checked with her if she could pack all of her things in one large bag and one carry-on roller bag. She confirmed with me that it would be no problem at all. In a way you could say that she exceeded her goal.

We flew first class and stayed at the amazing Waldorf Astoria in Maui. We met Ashley Wagner and Adam Rippon, two world class figure skaters that were on vacation there as well. We all hung out 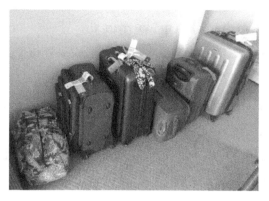 and drove the Hana Highway together to see some amazing waterfalls, cliffs, black sand beaches, and other natural beauties. We had relaxing days with fancy drinks followed by nice dinners with fancy drinks.

We hopped over to the Big Island next where we met another couple that was leaving and generously gave us all of their rum— SCORE! We did a helicopter tour over the volcanoes and waterfalls and even found our own private beach one evening. We were so happy that she was healthy for all of this. It seemed like luck. It was an amazing vacation and one I would reflect on during the challenges of the following year.

Not long afterward, we closed on a house in Northern Kentucky (NKY) and began the move. Though we had movers, Becca was not getting a lot of sleep and tended to stress about every aspect. During this transition, we were living apart for a few months as she worked from the OC and I lived in temporary housing in Cincinnati, returning to Wisconsin every other weekend. As we feared, she started getting sick. When I came home to help with the final move, she was miserably ill. I had envisioned us getting to the house, letting Becca recover, and taking our time with the unpacking process. She had other plans. Even if I could get her to let me do most of the work, she still had reports to complete for work and business travel planned.

After another tune-up, she became healthier but never fully recovered. By early October, we had a long weekend planned in Colorado with the Napa crew. As the time approached, she began to get sick again. I suggested skipping this trip to fully recover but she brushed it off knowing we would have a restful weekend in a scenic vacation house in the woods.

When we arrived at the airport I asked if her oxygen concentrator had already been shipped there or if it would arrive after we did. Seeing her response, I immediately realized that she had forgotten to order it. She reasoned that a couple of nights without it were no big deal. She would often skip nights during short travel weeks feeling it was not worth the effort. This was different, though. She was already ill and we were going to be at a much higher altitude.

"It's too late to order it anyway," she reasoned. Then her tough-guy attitude surfaced, "I'll just have to go a few nights without it." I grumbled at her with a clear "Hmmmmm." I gave her my stern disapproving look that almost certainly made her stop and reflect. Maybe we could try to order it the next day.

She felt terrible from the moment we landed and was laid out for the entire drive to the house. She was constantly in the back of my mind, as Mike and I sang along to 80s songs and discussed pulling a Thelma and Louise off the mountain road as a testament to our friendship. The idea was ultimately voted down by those riding in the back of the van, even though we had not really asked them.

Bec pretty much walked through the front door and went

straight to bed. Meanwhile, I caught up with our friend Meagan and her new man, fully prepared to give him a hard time. Now that he was hanging out with "the crew" he would have to deal with some good old fashioned harassment. I checked on Bec again before stepping outside to talk to Melanie and Stephanie while looking at the view. Her condition was a worry that beer and good conversation could not help me forget.

I got to bed a few hours later and could hear that her breathing sounded the worst that I had heard it. It was like amplified Rice Krispies. I kept telling myself that it was bound to get better, that she only needed a few good nights of sleep. She needed much more than that.

The next morning she slept in as well. I kept checking on her and really started to worry when we got back from hiking and she was not up yet. I helped her down the stairs and made a high calorie shake for her. We sat down to watch the football game and she was falling asleep between sips. After sixteen hours of sleep, if she could not keep her eyes open then something was seriously wrong. I searched for the nearest ER or urgent care clinic and found one a few miles away. I told her we were going and it was not up for discussion.

We walked in the door of a small urgent care clinic not far from the house. When they checked her oxygen level, it was 52 percent! Quick math tip: percent means "out of 100." They were shocked that she was even capable of standing there in front of them, much less having been able to walk in from the car. They immediately put her on oxygen and drew blood. When the results came back, they were not good. The doctor believed that she might be septic. This is a complication of an infection that can be life threatening. It took us both off guard as the doctor continued to explain that we would need to transfer to the hospital in Denver.

This was the first time I was seriously concerned whether or not she would survive a particular illness. In the past I had seen pneumonia lead to weight loss, exacerbations where she was exhausted and weak, fevers where her teeth chattered so loud I could hear it from across the room. But I had never worried whether or not she would recover. She had always recovered. That's what she did.

As we rode in the ambulance to the Denver hospital, I contemplated how she needed to stop working and focus on her health. I was not sure yet how I could convince her of that. As we drove, I gave the paramedics her mega-list of medications. I texted her mom and sister and explained the severity of her situation. While I did all of this, my mind kept slipping into worst-case scenarios.

Our long weekend stretched into a week as I found a local hotel from which I could walk to the hospital. The rest of my priorities would have to go on the back burner. My boss told me not to worry about a thing and just care for my wife. It seemed nice but would come back to bite me weeks later when he held me accountable for not catching a late shipment affecting my P&L (profit and loss).

Becca was admitted to the ICU so they could stabilize her. As she grew stronger, she would walk around this indoor track while monitoring her O_2 levels. It was a new experience watching her work this hard to do so little. She needed to get down to three liters of O_2

before they would let her fly home. We had another first as we went through the airport in a wheelchair. This first had some benefits when we were able to bypass long security lines and pre-board, but I would not recommend getting sepsis for more efficient travel.

After returning home, we started to plan her return to the hospital for the next day. However, after explaining her swelling to the doctor on-call, they wanted her to come in immediately. Her body was holding a lot of excess fluid which is a condition referred to as edema. It did not seem worrisome to deal with cankles for a few days, but her new Cincinnati doctors instantly became concerned with her heart. They instructed us to come in to the ER immediately. This kicked off another week in the hospital, but at least we were at home. It was at the conclusion of this hospital stay that we learned that she had experienced heart failure on the right side of her heart. Apparently, this was common with people with CF and other major lung problems. The heart had to do more work because the lungs were not effectively exchanging gases with the blood.

It was then that we had our first serious conversations about a double lung transplant. There was so much going on with her job and the holidays coming that she decided to start looking into it more seriously in January. In the meantime, she would go back to work. Only one more business trip was needed that year, and she agreed to utilize the wheelchair service. After that we would be ready for our annual Christmas visit to my sister Rachel's in Connecticut. Nothing too stressful in front of us and then it would be time to recover. I argued for a reduction to part-time work and for that too, she said that she would talk to her boss in January.

We were only a few weeks from a short vacation, reduction in hours, and being worked up for a transplant listing. I knew it would be a tough year for her health-wise but truly had no idea. She would never have that conversation with her boss and she would not be able to start the listing process in January. Her health had declined much more than we ever realized.

Even with the help of a wheelchair, business travel was tough. She needed to plan for the additional time and being ready early was not one of her strengths. There were points when she had to carry her bags and do other things that a lone traveler needs to do. By the time she returned, it was painfully clear to her that this could not continue indefinitely. She posted on the CF Facebook page to hear other stories but there were not many in her situation.

December 18, 2014: Becca's Post on CF page

Anyone here on 24/7 O_2 and still work full time? Anyone routinely travel for work with O_2? Just started on nearly 24/7 O_2 a few weeks ago and took my first trip for work with my POC (portable oxygen concentrator) this week. Exhausting and a real pain in the arse!! Contemplating how long this is going to be feasible…

She looked exhausted packing for Christmas at Rachel's house. I told her that we did not have to go. We could postpone the trip and plan it for when she was feeling better. She wouldn't have it. "I'll be fine. We're only going to relax around the house and I can catch up with my sleep there," she argued.

Aside from the haunting similarities with the Colorado trip in October, it made sense. We would have an oxygen concentrator and home IV antibiotics shipped to the house in Connecticut. By this point, Rebecca was on supplemental oxygen 24/7 and she struggled with stairs and any kind of mild physical exertion. The holiday was nice but we worried because the IV meds did not kick in like they usually did.

Our first Monday back to work and she called me at my office asking me to come home. I drove her into the hospital that night. As we sat in the waiting area, I suggested she post something on Facebook to tell her friends the latest. I knew the comments would provide some moral support. She had always kept her illness to herself and only started telling people about it in recent years. For most stays, she did not even tell her family that she would be inpatient, but she agreed to check in at the hospital.

December 29, 2014: Rebecca's Check in at the University of Cincinnati (UC)

Not exactly where I wanted to spend New Year's week, but at least I got to spend Christmas with family. #FUCF

In response to that post, she received seventy-two comments from friends and family wishing her well and telling her that they were praying for her. It was the response I had hoped for and she truly appreciated it. She would read through the comments and speak in amazement about how many people had responded telling me who said what. It lifted her spirits considerably.

The next day, she was working from the hospital while I worked from home. By the time we were both done, I told her I would come in. I was a little relieved when she told me that she wanted to go to sleep early. I would just come in on New Year's Eve and we could celebrate in her room.

CHAPTER 5

New Year, New Low

Unfortunately, our celebration would never happen. The next morning the doctor called with news of her decline and off to the hospital I raced with dread in the pit of my stomach. This was the timeframe where we had planned for her to shift to part-time, get listed, and fully recover from 2014. Was it already too late? I flashed back to October as I drove in wondering what was in store. The scary part was that unlike in Colorado, she had been sleeping, was a week into her antibiotic regimen, was utilizing supplemental oxygen, and had been under attentive care. If she was still declining, it would not be an easy fix.

I arrived in her room to see her with a BiPAP mask clamped around her mouth and nose. In addition to oxygen, this was providing extra pressure (bilateral positive airway pressure) so she did not have to work as hard to breath. It was not helping enough. I held it in place and fed her sponges of water when she asked for them. The medical staff was mainly talking to me because she was working so hard just to breathe. We discussed doing a bronchoscopy (bronch) which is a procedure during which they look into her lungs with a scope. They could also suction out some of the mucus. The pulmonologist felt that it might not be the best option at that time.

When they brought up intubation as a probable next step, it wasn't the procedure that scared me—it was the look of fear on Rebecca's face. They wanted to put a tube down her throat which was connected to a ventilator (vent). The idea was that the ventilator would do the breathing for her while she rested and recovered with the help of IV antibiotics. She would be sedated during the entire time she had the breathing tube down her throat. I understood what it was, but I did not know what it meant. I asked questions on side effects and ramifications but could not bring myself to ask the one main question I was thinking. What was her chance of survival? I was not ready to hear the answer and in the end, it did not matter whether I knew an exact percentage. This was her best chance, so the answer was simple.

She was someone who prided herself on how tough she was. I used to joke with her that she was the macho one, as she always played down any kind of procedure she required. Very few times had I seen her fearful, and this time the fear was very evident. I couldn't help but tear up myself as I worried that this would be the last time we would talk to one another.

The time for the procedure came quickly and I had to leave the room. I did not hear her weak voice say, "I love you." One of the doctors had to tell me she said it. "I love you, too," I said, trying to be loud enough for her to hear but not shouting it to the entire MICU. In a flash, I was out of the room. I had no time to think of any more questions, much less ask them. I knew we were in a good hospital that we had researched and I could see that the staff genuinely cared. I had to trust them to do their job.

It was a relief to take my mask off as the inside was damp with tears and snot. I dreaded what I had to do next, which was to call her parents. I did not have any conclusive information to tell them. I did not know if she was going to be okay, I did not know when to expect improvements, and I did not know if or when she would wake up. I just told them what I knew. Scott and Pete both asked if they should come out. I really could not answer that. I did not want to tell them to wait and risk her passing without them having had a chance to say good-bye. Brenda told me that she would come out when Becca was feeling better. She would wait until Bec woke up and they would decide on a date together. I felt like she did not fully understand the gravity of the situation, but I had explained it as best I could. I later found out that she had been sick and figured that maybe this factored into her reasoning. I set a goal for myself to keep everyone as informed as I could and let them know that they were welcome to come at any time. I extended this sentiment to all of her family.

I went back upstairs and the procedure was complete. She looked incredibly uncomfortable lying in that bed but she was unconscious. I sent out a text to our immediate family telling them what had been completed.

I stood in the corner of the room looking at her wondering how she would be able to cough up all of those secretions that were in her lungs. Then, she started coughing. Due to the tube down her throat, it was hauntingly silent. I could just see her go through the motions and make the facial expressions. She tried to sit up and cover her mouth but her hands were secured to the bed so she would not unknowingly pull out the tube. She coughed up a large amount of thick mucus which started coming out of her mouth. Her oxygen levels started to drop below 80 percent while I stood there frozen, not knowing what I should do. The respiratory therapist (RT) wiped it away with a towel then proceeded to suction her.

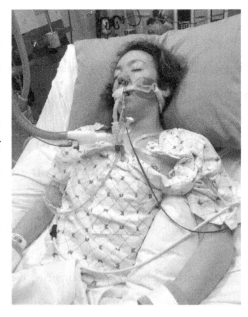

Suctioning was quite disturbing the first few times I saw it. There was a smaller tube that was inserted down the larger ventilation tube. When it was in far enough, she would involuntarily start to cough then they would press a button and it would open a connection to a vacuum system. As they held the button down and drew back on the smaller tube, I could see thick secretions being removed. As soon as it was out, her sats started climbing back to 100 percent. Both nurses and RTs would suction her whenever she needed to get something out which typically ended up being a few times per hour. A drop in sats would trigger an alarm which would alert her caregivers that she needed suctioning. As I sat in the room watching her numbers, I would step out and grab someone if they did not come quickly enough. Fortunately, they were very responsive. Each nurse had either one or two patients and there was a station right outside of her door.

I started thinking about how shitty things had become. I wished we were not here and did not have to deal with all of this. I thought back to better times, Hawaii, new homes, big moves...we had shared so much and I would not trade these memories for anything. I had always known that Rebecca was headed toward this point and the only way I could have avoided being there in that hospital room with her at that moment was if I was not with her. Our years together had been a blessing and what I really wanted was more time. In that moment I realized how fortunate I was to have all of these experiences, even if they led up to this. I was lucky to have had Rebecca in my life. As much as I hated what was happening, I appreciated what had brought me to this particular place. I suddenly felt thankful for all of the memories we created. And through the desire to want things to improve, I began starting every prayer with thanks, because I had a lot to be thankful for.

Lesson 4: Be thankful.

That thought did not make me feel good but it brought me a little peace. As I sat by her bedside, I smiled to myself about all of the unique memories and dumb stories we had amassed over the years. In addition to giving her many nicknames, one of which was Beccalicious, I also made up songs for her. I informed her that much like Fergalicious proclaimed in her song, Beccalicious was also "so delicious." So as I sat beside her bed, I softly sang "The Beccalicious

Song" for the first time that day…

> *"Her name is Beccalicious*
> *And she is so delicious*
> *She's Beccalicious so delicious*
> *Can't you see?*
> *She's Bec-ca Lee."*

It was a song to remind her of our normal life, of better days. If she was dreaming, I hoped that this would make those dreams happier. Coincidentally, it probably reminded her of how great of a singer-songwriter she married.

The next step for her caregivers was to insert a catheter (or foley) to capture and measure her urine output. Though sedated, she opened her eyes during the procedure and I could see her confusion. Before I could say anything, she sat up to give her male nurse a look and raise her restrained hands in a way of saying, "What the hell do you think you're doing!?" Fortunately, she believed me when I told her it was okay because she did not seem to accept his explanation. As she lay back down, she instantly fell asleep. I felt for her. She had that type-A personality where she always had a high level of control and understanding. But here she was, helpless. It was hard to look at her like that.

As the day dragged on, Rebecca would wake up periodically and try to communicate. She had this sense of urgency that made everyone nervous that there was something medically critical that we needed to know. I would pull out a pad and she would scribble illegibly while we would guess.

The nurse suggested I go home for the night and get some sleep but there was no way I could leave. Becca woke up and overheard this and asked me to stay. "Of course I'm staying," I told her. I wasn't going anywhere.

She instantly started to tear up out of guilt and then urgently needed to tell us something. It took ten minutes and a whole lot of scribbling to say that I should ask for a cot. There she was, sedated and intubated in the MICU and she was reminding me to ask for a cot. The last thing she needed to worry about was me being comfortable when she was going through all of this. It said a lot about who she was since she was in this position and thinking of my comfort first. I suppose it also suggested that she did not think I was bright enough to ask for one for myself.

They brought in a recliner and that was where I spent New Year's Eve: sitting in a recliner that would not stay reclined; fully garbed up and sweating profusely under my plastic gown, gloves, and mask; watching alarms and praying they were not of grave importance. I dozed off about ten minutes before the New Year and opened my eyes ten minutes afterward. Worst. New Year. Ever.

After a shitty, sweaty night's sleep, I woke up during a spontaneous breathing test. It was about 4:30 a.m. and they were messing with the ventilator. I was waiting for this since the day before because it would tell us if she could be extubated. She failed.

The test basically set the vent to mimic normal breathing

conditions aside from some higher oxygen concentrations. If she could keep her O_2 sats up above 90 percent then they could remove the tube. The simple work of using her diaphragm to expand her chest and pull in air was too much for her body to support and the last thing we wanted was to extubate her when she could not truly breathe for herself.

On New Year's Day 2015, I awoke still in the nightmare. The doctors would start rounds at 8 a.m. and I would have the chance to participate. They started with her background, "thirty-seven-year-old woman with end stage CF..."

End stage CF. It was the first time I had heard that in reference to my wife. I did not know the technical definition of that phrase but I was pretty sure I got the gist of it. They continued to discuss the case and I would ask for clarification when necessary but save most of my questions for the end. I wanted to make sure I understood what was happening, ask about alternatives, and be confident that she was getting the best care possible. I would not only ask questions, I would interject with my own observations when relevant. My contribution was my knowledge about her medical history and the play by play I could provide from the sheer number of hours I spent in the room. I was observant and could focus on nothing other than her condition.

I needed to be thinking critically during these discussions so I could do my part. I was not intentionally trying to avoid getting worked up or teary but I had my game face on and was trying to stay clear mentally. Focusing on performing my role was important because I felt I could add value to her care and be her voice. An emotional mess helped no one. I definitely did not want them to give me a sugar-coated version of reality. I also wanted them to know they could come to me and explain tough issues early and bluntly. When talking to the doctors, a critical part of advocating for her best care was asking good questions. These could help me to better understand her care and potentially identify symptoms or trends that provide diagnostic value.

Lesson 5: Ask a lot of questions and understand that you provide value even if you are not a medical expert.

I had a lot of questions, many of which I would ask her other caregivers over the course of the day. Asking the same question to everyone helped me gain a better understanding of what was happening, and if anyone was seeing things more optimistically or pessimistically than their colleagues. In order to understand our prospects I needed to know the meaning of all of the readouts on her monitor, key critical numbers, interpretation of test results, and reasons for ventilator setting selections. I learned a lot very quickly.

At the conclusion of rounds, I sent out a text update. It appeared that Bec might be on the vent for a day or two more but nothing was certain.

January 1, 2015 Group text: *She's doing ok now, they're thinking she can get off the vent tomorrow. This hospital has a good CF clinic and she is stable so we're optimistic on how the next day will go*

The plan was to slowly back off the vent support until she was at minimal settings. Once there, they would reduce her sedation and perform the spontaneous breathing test again. She was on propofol (for sedation) and fentanyl (a pain medication with sedative effects). She required much more sedation than would be expected for a person of her size. Perhaps this was because of her CF or maybe because she had reddish hair (we had heard at one point that this correlated to resistance to sedation). Whatever the reason, they continued upping her levels because she kept waking up and was too alert. They wanted her to be at a very specific sedation level. They should be able to wake her up and tell her what they are doing but she should basically stay asleep for the rest of the time. Her being too alert wasted precious energy so they wanted to keep it to a minimum. This was a constant struggle and discussion with her doctors.

One question I had was if they could increase her calories through the nasogastric tube (a feeding tube that went through her nose and down into her stomach). She was down to 95 pounds when she checked into the hospital and I knew she would need to gain some weight in order to qualify for a transplant. I had calculated the calories they were providing and it was only 1,600 calories a day. I asked to talk with the nutritionists but they were not there so I worked on the doctor and negotiated my way up to 1,950. I was ultimately shooting for 3,000 so I started my negotiations at 3,500. Through the next few discussions, we found agreement at 2,500 calories.

Right from the start, her RT asked that I not wake her up. Being alert can sometimes lead to panic and movement, which would lead to higher CO_2 levels in the blood and her levels were already high.

I could sit there holding her hand while talking quietly to her which was fine with me. It was emotionally exhausting when she woke and panicked or even just wanted to illegibly write something.

The RT was responsible for the ventilator, nebulized breathing treatments, and airway clearance. The airway clearance was critical and we had used varying methods throughout the years. Early on, we started with me pounding firmly on her torso using cupped hands to loosen the secretions so she could cough them up. A few years later, she was able to get a machine called The Vest (a high frequency chest wall oscillation device that filled with air and used pulsing pressure to help her dislodge and clear secretions). Some hospitals also had a percussor that she liked. This was a handheld device, with a contact area about the size of a palm that would pulse at a high frequency, much like the cupped hands technique.

Our RT told us about a bed that vibrated to perform airway clearance for someone on a ventilator with limited movement. Though it required maintenance, he called in a favor and his friend came in on his day off to fix it. It was one of the first instances where we saw her caregivers go above and beyond to care for her.

I snuck home for a quick shower and came back ready for the next night. I rebelliously slipped my arms out of the plastic sweaty gown and asked for an extra pillow. I was getting better at MICU life.

The next morning Bec began to stir and physically fight against her restraints. She would pull with her arms and kick her legs as she looked around confused. I would talk to her to try to calm her down but the nurse was much more successful because he had versed (another sedative) that he could push into her IV.

It was a new day and therefore, time for another—accurate, yet non-alarming—update.

January 2, 2015 Group text: *She got a little worked up this morning during her treatment but she's ok. Still waiting to talk to the Dr. about next steps.*

Twenty minutes later...

They need to do a breathing trial to determine if they can take her off the vent and because she was worked up her CO_2 levels didn't allow for the trial. Still waiting to discuss the plan

Twenty minutes later...

They are planning to do a bronch because it will clear mucus plugs and that's a potential cause of the CO_2. As a result she'll be on the vent for a few more days

This was rough news to take. We wanted to keep the number of days on the vent at a minimum so that her muscles did not atrophy too much and she could move around more and stir up secretions to be coughed out. But it was the only option at this point because her CO_2 levels, which should ideally be around 30 mEq/L, had risen to 90.

Bec opened her eyes to hear about the planned bronchoscopy and had to write something again. Over and over we tried to guess what her scribbles meant as she got more and more excited. She shook her head no and wrote with increasing urgency. The fact that she was ventilated and could not talk just added to the anxiety for everyone. It took about ten minutes for us to understand that she thought the plans for the bronch were a mix-up. She was remembering two days earlier when they said it was not necessary. At this point, I just wished she would stay asleep until she was healthier.

I had been pushing for her to get a bronch because she had been complaining that her lungs were so bad that she constantly felt like she was drowning. I hoped that they could pull out a lot of the secretions and she would be starting over with clearer lungs, which would be the boost she needed to get off of the vent. But after all was said and done, the bronchoscopy did not clear out the amount of secretions I had expected and her improvements did not come.

As the days passed, the more it seemed like we were just waiting for the other shoe to drop. The nurses warned me that many times they saw close family members get their own room in the ICU because they were not taking good care of themselves. I started going home at night because I came to a few realizations:

1. The hospital staff was skilled and responsive and they did not really need me there 24/7.
2. What I could add to the discussion during rounds was equally as valuable, even if I stepped out for a few hours.
3. I did not need to do *everything* that could potentially help; I had to look at the probabilities.

Sure staying the night might allow me to hear an alarm and pull someone in to help a minute sooner, but there was a good chance it would do nothing at all. It was not probable that I would affect any real change that night and I knew that I could not keep up a 24/7 watch for the long run.

Lesson 6: Sometimes the best way to take care of someone else is to also take care of yourself.

Though she would be a priority, I had to allow myself to come in second place. It meant stepping out of the room for lunch rather than eating protein bars in the room. It meant going home at night if there was nothing urgent or new.

My empty home was hauntingly quiet but at least it was home. It was nice to have a comfortable bed, but I would often lay there, unable to sleep. I'd scroll through my phone looking at pictures and re-watching videos I had taken of Rebecca. It felt a bit pathetic and clichéd like I was becoming Mel Gibson from *Lethal Weapon* (without the mullet), or maybe Van Damme from *Timecop* (who also had a mullet)…widowers living these lonely isolated lives, always looking backwards. I felt like things were going down a dark path but I couldn't get out of my own head. I started to imagine that this would be my future…minus the mullet.

CHAPTER 6

We're Not Alone

It had been just the two of us to this point but it was looking like family definitely wanted to come and see her. Her father texted, asking me about a good time to book a flight, while my sister and friend Meg were working with me on dates as well. After I updated the group on her dad's schedule, Brenda sent me a text telling me that she was coming and needed the name of the hospital and doctor. It would have been nice to coordinate dates but it was a minor issue at this point. I sent her the info and she sent me her itinerary.

> **January 3, 2015: Facebook post**
> *Not much news to report as they make some minor tweaks and watch her vitals which are stable. Her dad is arriving from Maine today and her mom will arrive on Monday. Becca's fighting!*

All was going well until Jessica texted me.

January 3, 2015 from Jessica: *Hey brother, I saw my mom is gonna be there Mon. When I talked to her last night she sounded like shit. She said she was sick and that the flu is going around where she lives. Can she get Beck sick?*

This was frustrating. I wanted to make everyone feel welcome and I knew this could potentially be a final visit but I could not expose Bec to something that dangerous. Doctors had determined that it was rhinovirus (the common cold) that pushed Bec over the edge to require a ventilator. Any additional respiratory illness could potentially kill her.

I was thankful to Jessica for being on top of this and she soon offered to call Brenda and follow up. The next thing I knew, Brenda was calling me. She told me that she just had a cold and that Jess was blowing it out of proportion. I was in a very awkward situation but I told her that I was sorry and she could not come. Even if she just stayed at the house she could get me sick and if I developed symptoms, I would not be able to go see her myself. I had even started taking a daily zinc supplement because I feared catching a cold and leaving Rebecca with nobody in the room to talk to her or advocate for her. There was no way I would expose Bec to that, even if Brenda really wanted to see her.

That same day, Scott arrived from Maine. My first priority was to prepare him for what he was about to see. I used the ride from the airport to warn him about the things that alarmed me: hand restraints, alarms, and most importantly, the sight of her. When we arrived at the hospital, I let him have some time in the room by himself so he could talk to her and have some privacy. When I did come in, I explained what the pumps were for, what all of the monitors meant, which numbers were most critical, and what we could do about it.

I had been asking a lot of questions and encouraged him to do the same. A big part of my focus was to try to be a support to him. It

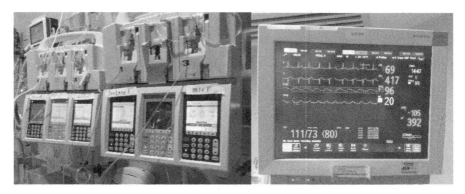

was hard for both of us, but I was more used to dealing with it. I had found that when I provided updates to people, explained the care plan, what we were hoping to see, and any positive changes she had shown, it was comforting to me as well.

Rebecca had a breathing tube down her throat and a feeding tube through her nose. She did not look comfortable. Her pulmonologist approached us about placing a PEG tube (percutaneous endoscopic gastrostomy) or G-tube. This is a flexible feeding tube placed through the abdominal wall allowing nutrition to be pumped directly into her stomach.

Before she got sick, she had been planning to get one to help her increase her weight so she could qualify for a transplant and I was up for anything that would make her more comfortable. The problem was that the gastrointestinal (GI) team disagreed with the ICU team and did not want to do the procedure. When the GI team came down to discuss it with me, they rolled in five deep. Their attending (the head physician) explained to me that they felt Bec may not want the procedure because of what she had said during her last appointment.

"She definitely wants the tube. She told me recently," I said.

The attending then explained that Bec had so many stomach issues that it would make more sense to wait and resolve those issues before moving forward with stomach surgery. I leveled with them, "For the past five years, Rebecca has gone to several different GI doctors in the hopes that they could resolve the issues. Despite all of the different work ups, they have not been able to. I hope that your team will be able to figure it out but I don't want to let that be the deciding factor on whether or not she gets this procedure. If it hasn't been resolved in the past few years, I'm not convinced that you can resolve it in the next week."

That pretty much stopped the full court press and they left to consider it. Our pulmonologist was pushing hard for it and I got the sense that if they would not do it, he would find somebody who would. The decision came back and we got it scheduled. The procedure itself was quick. When they wheeled her out I called AT&T to increase my text plan because all of the updates I'd been sending had already pushed me over. They performed the procedure and brought her back to the room, and I was still on the phone. I am not sure if that speaks well for the hospital or just poorly for AT&T, but in either case she was back.

Soon after, the nurse knocked on the door and told me that I had visitors. I was confused because we had just moved to Cincinnati and none of our friends or family were closer than a five-hour drive.

"There is a couple, Gio and Sylvia, in the waiting room," he told me. I could not believe it. I used to work with Gio in Connecticut and we moved out to Wisconsin at the same time. He and his wife had just driven seven hours to show their support.

They said I did not have to step out if I was busy. They drove all this way for a just a *chance* of having a cup of coffee with me. They were not without their own family health challenges either, which made it more impressive. It was one of the nicest gestures I had ever experienced. With Scott sitting in the room with Becca, I felt I

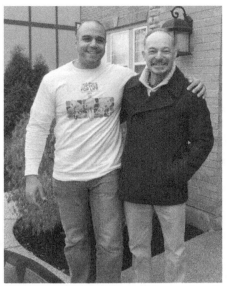

could step out and show them our new home in Northern Kentucky. It was the first break and a bright spot in a pretty dark month.

When Scott left I felt bad that he did not see her wake up and get off of life support. Little did I realize that we had plenty more time in front of us on that ventilator. Once he left, a quiet house got quieter and I went back to my normal hospital routine. I sat in the room holding her hand. I would sing songs quietly while I surfed the web. Sometimes, I found it hard to look at her in that condition all day long so I would move to the recliner where I could not see her face.

I found my mind constantly drifting back to worst case scenarios. I would think about the logistics of the funeral. I would imagine having to find a plot in Connecticut like she had wanted. I thought about trying to move on with my life and what I could do next. I was constantly battling with myself and trying to get these thoughts out of my head. I knew that even if the odds were against us, nothing was set in stone. In the end, I tried to use some logic. I needed to have something I could fall back on to remind me of where my thoughts should be focused.

There was no benefit in thinking these thoughts. If I lost her I would be miserable. If I thought about this day after day beforehand and then lost her, I would be just as miserable. There's no "getting a jump start" on the mourning process. I was also not going to be any more shocked if I did not dwell on the negative. I knew it was a possibility. I was not making any future scenario easier by making myself more miserable in the present. So why torture myself? She was still alive.

Lesson 7: Do not mourn for somebody who is alive.

Good logic, but if I was not careful, those thoughts would drift back in again. I had to tell myself that I would worry about that if and when it was necessary. I had to actively work to keep the perspective I was determined to maintain. I could make the decision but the challenge came with actually stopping the runaway train that was my thoughts.

The best thing I could come up with in dealing with the situation without her was to know that I was not without her. When I saw something funny, I would take a snapshot and text it to her phone (like when her heart rate was 69). I would talk to her when I was in the room and tell her she was doing well. My standpoint was that she could read it *when* she woke up. I also focused on the fact that Rebecca had been able to recover from quite a bit when she had sufficient sleep. Right now, her body was getting a much needed rest.

I was looking forward to our next visitors which would be Jessica, her boyfriend Trey, and Becca's stepdad Pete. I did my best to prepare everyone for what they would see, the same way I did for Scott. It was understandably tough for Pete and he could not spend long periods of time in the room. He and Trey would step out for periods during the day and return later. He was angry that this had to happen to Becca, but was adamant that the doctors did not know how much of a fighter she was. He was right about that.

Jessica handled things better than I expected. It was the two of us in the room most of the time. We joked around and told Becca stories. There was a positive atmosphere as we joked around sitting on either side of the hospital bed. We had some good conversations during this time. I stressed that we could not compare her current state to the previous year, we needed to compare with the previous day. And if we had a bad day, sure we would take it on the chin. But if the next day brought improvements we needed to recognize them. I preferred to focus on little improvements at this time rather than how far she needed to go to fully recover. I remember making the point to her, "If today is better than yesterday, we're doing okay." It drove home another lesson.

Lesson 8: Two steps forward and one step back is still an improvement.

Pete took us out to a nice dinner. Jess cleaned the house. It was a tough time but we were in it together. We watched and waited through the daily ups and downs with no real understanding of what to expect next.

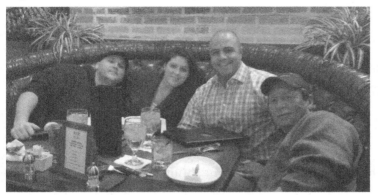

Left to right: Trey, Jessica, Ray, Pete

We were often all in the room, for rounds. The morning brought a new attending physician who was much more pessimistic about Rebecca's direction. She made it clear that the lack of improvement suggested that Bec was not likely to recover. It was the news that always seemed to be one update away, that unspoken threat. It happened quickly and when she was gone, Jessica looked at me and asked if she said what she thought she said. I nodded. All I could do was put my hand on her shoulder for a second then let her process it. It was the worst news we had received to this point and it hit everyone pretty hard. A long quiet morning followed as we sat there trying to sort this out in our heads. Maybe this doctor was just more pessimistic. Maybe Bec would start a turnaround since her numbers had been consistent for a few days.

That afternoon, the mood improved a bit when the attending

returned with a new theory. Maybe she was not in such bad shape. With all of her edema, it was clear she was retaining fluids. Doctors had told us that it was not problematic, only cosmetic but she felt differently. This fluid could be increasing pressure outside her lungs as well as saturating them. Perhaps she could improve once this was flushed from her system.

Bec had checked into the hospital at 95 pounds. Throughout all of this, she was only getting tube feedings and her muscles were atrophying so her *real* weight must be less. However, she was holding so much water that her weight reached 142 pounds. She was almost unrecognizable. Her hands were so puffy it was like she was wearing mittens. When I looked at her, I found myself focusing on these three freckles under her left eye just to recognize her.

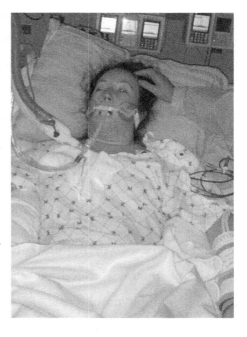

She would be diuresed, or given furosemide to help her pee off this excess fluid she had retained. I suggested a few shots of espresso added to the tube feed to work in concert with the furosemide but apparently that was not how they did things in Cincinnati…or in hospitals.

They also found that she had cultured new bacteria and added a new antibiotic to her regimen. We had a plan. This helped her string together a few good days in a row and by the time her family was leaving she was showing consistent improvements.

On the final morning of their visit, Bec's nurse held us to the policy of only letting two of us in her ICU room at a time. Unsure of why this was, we came to find out that she aspirated during the night. They believe she had basically vomited into her lungs. I could see that her vent support, pressure and oxygen percentage, was much higher and her sats were on the low end. This meant she was getting more help yet doing worse; it was a notable setback. She was so fragile at this point that she would actually desat when they turned her slightly to change her position. She would soon be diagnosed with aspiration pneumonia and the second group of visitors would have to leave on a bad note. It was a rough day.

I was raised Catholic and was always good at making it to church…on Christmas. Despite less than perfect attendance, I tried to maintain a line of communication to the Man upstairs. During this ordeal, I sometimes found myself praying every few minutes and definitely multiple times a day. Her grandmother Kate, my mother, her friend Cynthia, and several others all had her on their church's prayer lists. My mother had always stressed that when more than one person prays to God for something, the prayer is more powerful.

I saw Facebook comments stream in after each of my daily updates on her page and it made me feel better to know that there were others out there praying for her as well. Now that I was spending my nights at home, I had extra time on my hands to worry about what was happening in the hospital. I could not fill that time with booze because I knew that at any minute, I could get a call and need to drive in to the hospital. I decided to fill it with a combination of thinking, praying, and Facebook. It was only natural that at some point, I would combine these. I was a member of a CF Facebook page and thought it would be a good place to share our story.

January 6, 2015: Post to the CF page

My wife Rebecca is 37 and has CF. We've been together for 17 years this month (married 11). Unfortunately in 2014 her health declined significantly despite her consistent efforts in doing her treatments, going to the Dr., and getting her rest. She checked into the hospital on Monday 12/29 then experienced "respiratory failure" and was moved to the MICU where we spent New Year's Eve with Becca sedated and on a ventilator. I've been involved with volunteering with the CFF and Bec's been involved with surviving. Basically, we do what we can.

We've had an amazing outpouring of well wishes and support from friends and family for which I'm SO thankful. There are so many ups and downs with this disease...but now I'm just asking for some prayers and well wishes for an amazing person and the toughest fighter I know...Beccalicious, Becca Lee, Sugar Plum, Sugar Spice, and Super Chunk...and a dozen other names I have for her! Thanks in advance.

The fact that this got over 500 likes and almost 170 comments provided a certain feeling of support. We were part of a community. The positive comments were encouraging and it felt less like asking for sympathy and more like asking for support because these people understand the struggle so well. Back in the room, I would watch the responses flow in all day long. The online CF community is strong partially because it is the safest. There are limited face-to-face interactions due to the high risk of spreading infection. Additionally, there are only about 30,000 people in the US with the disease making it incredibly isolating.

There was also a negative side to this. There are so many who are taken by the disease and being online, we saw a lot of postings. In some cases, they were people with whom we had communicated. Even though we had not met them in person, it was disheartening to experience this loss. However, in spite of this, there were people available who understood and shared their experiences. It provided hope for recovery and eventual transplantation.

Around the ten-day mark, when the pulmonologist spoke to me about doing a tracheotomy (trach) the feedback from the page cited firsthand accounts and encouragement that this was a good idea. It was a helpful tool to keep things in perspective. Her doctor told me that studies showed this was her best chance of survival. She would be on the ventilator for a while longer and it would allow them to drop her sedation. She would also be much more comfortable. It was scary to imagine them cutting a hole in her neck and running the ventilator tubes in from there rather than through her mouth, but the risks were relatively low. The best part was that they could then drop her sedation and she could be awake on the vent!

"You had me at 'awake,' doctor!" I told him. Okay, I did not say that but I definitely would have had I thought of it then. He explained how the scar would not be too noticeable and it would heal up quickly. I did not care about that at all. There was a chance that Bec could wake up and I could not wait!

It took a few days to schedule but once it was done she looked so much more comfortable. I could see it in her expressions and in the way she lay in the bed. By this point, she was recovering from the aspiration and morning was coming. I could not wait for her to wake up.

Amid the medical decisions, I had to start Rebecca's disability claim for her job. I called and answered all of the questions to get this set up. Not long afterward I received a phone call from the insurance company calling to talk to Bec. I explained how she was in a chemically induced coma on a ventilator but that I could answer the questions since I was the one who filed the claim. Without a power of attorney, they could not talk to me about the case I filed. We had signed one many years earlier but there was no way I could find it in our new house. I was told that they could not discuss the case with me but if I called and provided an update, they could use the information.

So every couple of weeks, I would call up and talk. It seemed a bit ridiculous. Any feedback I wanted, would have to come through her company's human resources (HR) department. It was good that I had that number because I was soon going to need it. I did not think much of it when the MICU social worker came to Rebecca's room. As I looked at her expression, I quickly realized that something was wrong.

"Rebecca's insurance has termed," she told me. Wait, what was that supposed to mean? I stumbled through a response asking her if that meant terminated and she confirmed. I knew she was still employed and it must be a mistake, but I also knew that if something went wrong in the insurance department, it would bankrupt us and ruin Rebecca's hopes for a transplant. This happened at 6 p.m. on a Friday.

At the time, it felt like the world was collapsing. Becca was still recovering from an aspiration and in terrible shape and now we could be facing a bill large enough to bankrupt us. It felt like things could not get worse, and then they got a little better. She had a good weekend. She climbed back to minimal vent support and had no major instances.

The following Monday, after not worrying about it at all, I connected with her HR. As it turned out, her company had changed their insurance carrier from Cigna to Aetna and she just had a new policy. I felt like I had just dodged a bullet. A few phone calls later and we had all of the information the hospital required. Suddenly, the whole world looked a little brighter.

Lesson 9: Understand that things may not be as bad as they seem in the moment. Give it time.

As I reflected on this, our struggles to have children came to mind. If we had been successful in starting a family as we had wanted so badly, I would have an eight-year-old during all of this—a child that I would need to care for, explain things to, and drive to school. This would have been incredibly challenging throughout the current situation, in a new town with no friends or family nearby. At the time, it was incredibly disappointing that we could not have kids. This one shift in our reality changed my perspective completely.

CHAPTER 7

I'm Coming Out

Meanwhile, I was looking forward to the next visitors, Rachel and Meg. They had both been so supportive with all of their calls and offers to visit. They would arrive soon, Rachel from Connecticut and Meg from North Carolina. Timing was tight for both of them because they worked full time so they would only have a couple of days but they were supporting me and following Rebecca's progress as closely as anyone.

Two days before their arrival, Brenda called. She got right down to it, "I'm coming out."

Hearing about the aspiration, she decided that it was time. I asked her point blank, "Are you still sick?"

"I'm not sick. I was never sick. I just had some allergies and a little cold at the end," she told me.

As I define it, "a little cold" means "sick" but aside from that, she had already admitted to being sick and she was changing her story. If she just said she was better I would have accepted it but knowing she was spinning I wondered how could I trust her? I told her if she was still sick it was going to put me in a difficult situation because I could not let her into the room. The truth of the matter was that I was not going to let anything risk Rebecca's recovery.

She told me that she could get a doctor's note. I told her not to worry about it but I said that if she was sick when she arrived, she could not go in. She went on to explain that she had allergies and that she would probably be sniffling from our cats. Then she told me that she had a smoker's cough, which I didn't know was even a thing. I mentioned that Rachel and Meg would be out over the weekend and she snapped back quickly "What's that supposed to mean?!" Her aggression took me back a little. I had been hosting all of the visitors for Rebecca while taking care of her daughter, keeping her updated. Perhaps she was angry that she had to cancel her first trip.

"I just want you to be aware that they've been planning to be here and that there are only two visitors allowed in the room at a time." I figured the risk for overlap was low because they would be arriving in two days and their visit was short.

When I got off the phone I could not shake the thought that she would be blowing her nose and coughing so there would be no symptoms that I could use to determine if she was really sick. I called her back and apologetically asked her to get the note. I was not really sure how they could confirm there was no illnesses in a quick visit but I would always regret it if I did not do everything I could. The note came in a few hours and did provide me some relief.

When she emailed me her itinerary, I found that she had booked a flight arriving late the next night. This meant she would arrive just before Rachel and Meg. An added surprise was that she apparently planned to stay for two full weeks. I reasoned that it was a tough situation where things were changing quickly. Maybe she was worried that she would not see her daughter again. She may have just overlooked telling me about the length of her stay. We would make it work.

The rest of her family had thanked me for being there for Rebecca and some even commented that she was lucky to have me. Brenda mostly asked for updates and details and aside, from a "ty" in a text, she did not show much appreciation or interest in how I was doing. This was okay because everyone handles these situations differently. In some ways, I was looking forward to her visit. She would better understand what Rebecca and I had been dealing with for years and how I was on top of her care. Even if it was not her way to express appreciation, she would see that her daughter was in good hands. I could not imagine it doing anything but helping our relationship in the long run.

As I drove her back from the airport, I began preparing her for what she would see. I did not get very far. She asked about Becca's sedation and I explained that she was on versed and fentanyl drips, which are amounts slowly but constantly infused. Before I could finish my sentence, she cut in asking why they were not using propofol. Before I could fully answer that, she jumped in asking about fentanyl, then about why they were using more than one medication.

I tried to continue responding patiently, but when she started getting annoyed at the answers and cutting me off with increasing attitude I became frustrated. At the point when she started lecturing me that the doctors were giving her too much sedation, she had barely let me answer any of her questions. I jumped in fairly annoyed at this point and said "LOOK, if you want me to answer your questions you're going to have to let me finish a sentence!" We were off to a fantastic start.

Aside from the courtesy thing, I was frustrated because she did not even know the dosages or the specifics of what was happening, yet she was telling me what Bec's treatment should be. I had been living this day in and day out for weeks, talking in detail with her caregivers almost every hour. If I could be patient enough to try to answer her questions, she could be patient enough to listen to the answers.

I went on to explain how we had gotten to her current sedation regimen and what medical changes had driven each decision but that did not matter. It turned out that Brenda had seen somewhere online that hospitals were awarded points for keeping patients sedated for longer than was required. Somehow points equaled money so because of this, hospitals kept many patients sedated unnecessarily. She detailed her conspiracy theory, while I winced inside all the while.

I explained that this was a good hospital with capable doctors that we had researched before moving out. I had been working closely with all of her doctors who truly cared for Rebecca and wanted her to recover. After weeks in the MICU, the last thing I wanted to hear was an unsubstantiated claim that her doctors had it out for her.

Living so far away, it was easy to distrust doctors she had not met—easier than accepting Rebecca's current condition. The best solution I could come up with was to encourage her to ask a lot of questions during the rounds. I told her not to leave anything unsaid if it concerned her and that she might have a question that I had forgotten to ask. If she would not listen to me, she could ascertain for herself. When we made it to rounds, she asked none of those questions. This was fine because she was either starting to understand that Rebecca was receiving good care or she felt her theories were not worth discussing. In either case, it was not on me to try to rebut them during a frustrating discussion. This concern was hers alone and I did not need any more worries.

Lesson 10: Do not take the worries of others onto your own shoulders.

Back in the room, I offered to step out and give her some alone time with Rebecca but she did not need it. I explained much of the equipment and readouts to her because the room could be overwhelming. Then, I showed her the pad where Bec had written *Did you call my mom?* on New Year's Eve, so she would know Bec thought of her.

I took some time to explain the importance of the saturation levels with respect to her ventilator settings. It had various ways to support her by expanding her lungs with pressure, increasing the oxygen up to 100 percent (room air is around 20 percent), dictating the length of her exhale, and determining a minimum number of breaths per minute. These functions impacted her O_2 and CO_2 levels significantly. So when she was getting less pressure support and less oxygen (minimal settings), if her oxygen saturation was close to 100 percent most of the time, it was a good day. My morning training session had stretched to an hour by this point.

When Rachel arrived, Brenda did not provide the warmest reception but when Meg arrived she was downright rude. Brenda had returned from getting a coffee and a face to face, "Hello, Brenda" from Meg was met with silence as she walked by and sat down.

We all looked at each other a bit surprised then Rachel said, "Brenda, you remember Meg, right?" It was at that point that I realized that she saw them as competition for a space in the room. So instead of being happy that Rebecca had this support from people who loved her, she was annoyed that they were there. She would only have to deal with them for two days then she would remain in town for another twelve so I was not sure why there was such an issue. I decided to implement a shift system where the girls would swap out with me and Brenda for two hours at a time. I gave Brenda first choice of the shifts as well.

After a string of good days, they were able to reduce Becca's sedation and we were soon waiting for her to wake up. This was thrilling as we all waited for her to open her eyes. It would be a few days before she comprehended anything because of the time and volume of sedation she had received.

In her first shift, Brenda told me flat out that if Rebecca woke up, she was not going to leave the room and that she "trumped" the girls. I did not tell her that if I was willing to step out, she would need to as well. In one of my wiser moments, I did not respond at all.

At the end of Rachel's last night we stopped home for a quick bite to eat while Brenda stayed in the room. I also had the chance to get in a quick workout. I figured with all of the anxiety and frustration, I would get on that treadmill and just take off...running in grand fashion...leaving all of that stress behind. As I ramped up the speed it became increasingly clear that this was not going to be the intense movie sprinting scene I had imagined. After a month of holiday eating and a few weeks of this hell, my cardio was the first to take a hit. It made me recognize that I needed to start making exercise more of a priority.

Meanwhile, Brenda ended up getting almost four hours in the room but texted me every time they made her step out. When we returned she said she was "in there for only ten minutes," which was an exaggeration compared with the texts she had sent and what I had experienced with those same medical interruptions. When the time came, I had to make it clear that Rachel *would* get some privacy to say good-bye. This was an important part of everyone's visit because you never knew if this was the last time they would see Rebecca. At this point, I was just looking for this unnecessary drama to end. And after all of the battles for time in the room, as soon as Meg left Brenda went down to the lobby to sit in a more comfortable chair and stayed there for a few hours.

As I sat in Bec's room looking around, my tension level dropped and things started to seem a little funnier to me. The humidifier on the ventilator caught my eye.

January 18, 2015: Facebook post

The humidifier instructions on Bec's ventilator say she should read a book and have a glass of wine…but don't have 2.

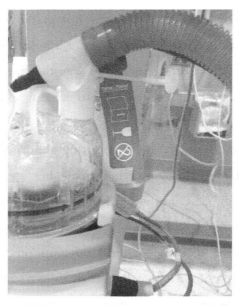

Rebecca may not have followed all of the instructions, but at least she did not exceed the allowable amount of wine. Then, as quickly as my tension level dropped, it rose again. They needed to increase the sedation again due to her rising blood pressure. They believed that Becca had some kind of anxiety issue as well as some addiction to the narcotics she was receiving, and they needed to wean her off of them more cautiously.

Another bronch followed and then there was a surprisingly quick decline in her condition. Suddenly her CO_2 level passed 100 mEq/L, which was a dangerous sign that her lungs were not functioning well. An increase in CO_2 drives a drop in blood pH and hers reached 6.8 (normal blood pH level is 7.35 to 7.45). The MICU fellow (a physician in a medical training period called a fellowship) told us that Rebecca was fighting the vent. I understood this to mean that she was trying to breathe at the pace that SHE wanted. That sounded exactly like Bec.

After discussing this with the attending physician, he returned more pessimistic than before. He told us that in order to stop Becca from fighting the vent, they would need to administer a paralytic. This basically prevented her from being able to move at all. Because it would be terrifying to wake up unable to move, they would also increase her sedation.

They attached a sensor to her forehead and a bunch of wires to her scalp to monitor her brainwaves so that they would not over-sedate her. This made the already overwhelming arrangement of equipment even more intimidating. In addition to new outputs on the first monitor, they brought in a second monitor with more readouts.

When they administered the paralytic, her oxygen saturation began to drop. As they bagged her, her sats continued to drop. One respiratory therapist called in the fellow while the other bagged her. The alarm triggered before the calls for help got louder and soon they were yelling into the MICU for help. Nurses and doctors raced into the room as her sats plummeted from 90s to 80s to 70s to 60s. They continued to drop, even with all of the work the staff was doing. They switched to a new oxygen source while someone else ran for a new ventilator.

We stood there in the corner. I had my arm around Brenda. She said she couldn't watch and left for all of ten seconds before coming back. At one point I looked above the bed and wondered if Becca's spirit was there hovering. It seemed like this was where it would end for her, for us. I thought back to how I had imagined our last moments and it was not like this. As I'm sure most do, I imagined a quiet hospital room with both of us able to say a few last words to each other. I imagined a certain level of peace and acceptance as she faded away. I definitely did not expect the chaos of a crammed ICU room with people yelling and racing against the clock.

It was somewhere in the 50s when her sats stopped dropping. Then they crept up a percent or two. Then they crept up a few more…it soon became a slow climb back into the 90s. What the hell had happened!? They thought it might be the vent so they swapped it out but eventually concluded that when she fully relaxed, she lost the positive end-expiratory pressure (PEEP) in her lungs. Basically, the air sacs closed up. It took time and pressure but they were able to correct it. I updated the rest of the family, trying not to alarm them, knowing the danger had passed.

January 20, 2015 Group text: *Bec's ok…but her pH dropped too low because she is still not in sync with the vent. They needed to give her something to temporarily control her breathing and right after her oxygen dropped quickly but they got her back up. They're not sure but think it was a problem with the vent.*

They changed settings on the vent in an attempt to help her expel the extra CO_2. It was getting late but we were not leaving until it started changing direction. Every half hour brought new results. Most were no better than the last. Finally it started to improve. Exhausted, we left for home. During the car ride, Brenda said something that would stick with me, "Does Rebecca have a will?"

I told her *no*, but that we had discussed a few of her personal goods. As we continued to drive I started to think: Does she expect to get something valuable if Becca passes? We had planned our finances *with* one another. Would I have to deal with a funeral and her mother trying to claim a car, some of my furniture, or half of my remaining savings? It seemed ridiculous to consider but as much as I pushed that thought away, it would creep back in.

The next day, Rebecca was continuing to maintain a poor, but good enough CO_2 level in the 80s. They expected to keep her on the paralytic for two days total and we were just holding our breaths that nothing got worse. With regard to her long-term prognosis, we knew that she would need a transplant as soon as she was healthy enough. I had started looking at a few programs but many would not list a patient if they had been on a ventilator for more than a few days. At this point, it had been almost three weeks.

During the previous day, they told us that she would not likely be able to breathe without the support from a ventilator while she still had these lungs. It took a while to wrap my head around this. We not only needed to find a hospital that would transplant a patient that had been on the vent for a while, but they needed to transplant her *from* the vent.

Suddenly, the get well soon sentiments did not seem appropriate. Rebecca was not going to simply recover and she was not going to be extubated with these lungs—maybe not ever. Her lungs were truly end stage and they were taking Bec with them. Her only shot was a transplant and that was becoming less likely by the day. If this was true, what did I have to hope for, what was the plan? With Rebecca so sick, all I could focus on was whether each day was better than the day before and pray for one more chance to talk with her.

January 19, 2015 Group text: *Bec's lung function hasn't improved for a while and they feel she could be on the vent longer than we had hoped. She may need to stay on it until she gets her transplant. We're hoping to talk to the CF doctor soon and learn more about how that would work.*

The next shoe dropped very quickly after that when they told us that she would probably not qualify for a transplant because she was too sick. Our Hail Mary was no longer realistic. I naturally tried to think of what the best case scenario would be, but there was no escaping the logic. If both of these statements were true, then Rebecca would remain on a ventilator until she passed with no chance of getting transplanted. It was maddening knowing that her lungs were the problem but she could not receive new lungs because the old ones were so bad. I struggled with the wording when I sent out the next text. I was intent on telling the full truth but it helped no one to be an alarmist.

January 21, 2015 Group text: *Bec's settling into her new settings. More swollen today as they try to let her pee off some excess fluid. CF doctors are saying she probably won't qualify for a transplant so we're looking to get the most out of these lungs.*

I struggled to derive a new plan. We needed to hope for something and it was Jessica who called with an idea. Trey's sister worked at Barnes Jewish Hospital in St. Louis, one of our top choices for transplant hospitals. The idea was for her to get Rebecca accepted as a patient by their lead pulmonologist. If she was a patient there, it had to help her chances at transplantation.

Jess proceeded to forward everything that Google had to offer. She was convinced that once Becca was transferred there, they would be able to help her recover better than in Cincinnati. She was also expecting an improved chance of being listed if Bec was a patient. I tried to manage her expectations. The facts of her condition were not changing. It was not like she had an unconfirmed diagnosis, she had been seen by over a dozen different doctors. We had also researched UC before moving out and I saw firsthand that they were providing great care.

I called our insurance company and did some research on the transport process. Since she was not listed yet, the transfer would be discretionary. This meant that we would likely have to pay for the transport. Due to her condition and the distance, she would have to be transferred via a medical flight with an estimated cost of around $50,000.

Not only was this an excessive bet against the odds, but it did not include any costs we might incur during or after the transplant. As it was, I had not been to work in weeks and my vacation time was running out. I had been at the job for less than a year and did not qualify for the Family Medical Leave Act (FMLA), if that even applied to me. Rebecca was receiving some disability pay, but it was a huge gamble—a gamble that could bankrupt us, or me.

At minimum, I needed enough money to cover her insurance premiums, the mortgage, and food. I was not ready to rule it out but I needed more evidence than an impressive bio for some pulmonologist. I boiled it down to one main question, "Will transferring her there improve her chances at getting listed, enough so that it would be likely?"

By the time we had our meeting with her CF doctor (Dr. Patricia Joseph) I was expecting that this was probably not going to be a good option. Aside from everything else, she just did not appear well enough to survive the trip. We sat down in the consultation room and Dr. Joseph responded to us as I had expected. She said that a transfer would probably not increase her chances to get listed. She said that they would be happy to continue to care for Bec but it was ultimately our decision. We had her forward Becca's file to the pulmonologist at Barnes Jewish to see if it was even an option. Even if he would consider taking her case, the transfer seemed unlikely but I decided I would let it play out for Jessica's sake.

As the conversation shifted to her care, Dr. Joseph was straightforward as I hoped she would be, though she said what I had hoped she wouldn't. She was surprised Rebecca had survived as long as she had. Normally when CF sufferers in Bec's condition are intubated, they survive for a few days then secretions begin to pool, carbon dioxide levels rise, blood pH drops, and they can no longer maintain oxygen levels. Her prognosis was grim. It was likely that Bec had "days to weeks" to live. There was likely no transplant in her future and no Hail Mary.

I really just wanted her to wake up, but then I dreaded any pain or fear that came with being awake. In the end, there was nothing I could do but more of the same. I would still come in, hold her hand, and sing "The Beccalicious Song." I wanted to make sure she was comfortable but the rest was out of my hands.

We went back to the room to find another doctor evaluating her. Her bladder pressure had spiked. The fluids she had been retaining had caused an increased her internal organ pressures. He told us that if we could not bring them down, they would have to make a cut down her torso to let her body expand thereby reducing the pressure. They would cover her body with plastic to hold everything in place.

We had just returned from a discussion where they told us she was not going to make it and now there was a chance that in her last days, she would be cut completely open. All I could think was that if she was not going to make it, then I prayed it happened soon so she did not have to experience any of this pain. As with everything else, getting past this was about rolling with the punches. When it came down to what we could do, it was all about reducing the pressure. They pumped her stomach, performed an enema, gave her furosemide for the fluid retention, and we waited. The pressure went up again. As the stomach pumping and diuretic continued, we prayed that we would reach a reversal point. Finally, the numbers started to creep down a little at a time. Once they reached the safe zone we headed home, feeling beat up after one of the toughest days yet.

Brenda wanted Becca's sister to come out but Jessica was still hanging on to the possibility of a transfer to St. Louis. She told Jess that she had a private consultation with Dr. Joseph (aside from our discussion) and was told more dire news. I strongly suspected that this never happened but I also knew why she lied. She wanted to appear as the authority to convince Jess to come out without a long discussion. She basically told her that Bec would not make it another day or two, which was not far from the doctor's prognosis. I tried not to get too annoyed at her story and reminded myself that everyone deals with these situations differently and that she loves her daughter and was trying to control the situation in the only way she knew how. We both wanted Jess to come out but approached it differently.

Immediately after their quick conversation, I spoke to Jess and clarified the prognosis. We spoke for almost two hours as I told her that St. Louis was probably not going to work out. She had a tough time accepting that because it represented giving up on the only hope we had for survival. I wanted her to be there as well because I knew that is what Bec would have wanted.

The one thing that got me going on tough days was the fact that Bec had always told me, "I want you to be there when I die." I knew that could be at any point. On my toughest days, I reminded myself that I HAD to be there. Even if she did not know, I had to be there. It was one of the most important promises I made to her. I also knew she would want her sister there too if she could. I finally convinced Jess by saying that if for some reason we started to transport Bec to St. Louis while she was driving, I would call her and tell her to turn around. Worst case, she would just do a little more driving that day. She agreed and there was never a reason to call.

A few hours after she arrived, we were sitting in the hospital room. Bec had shown some signs of improvement and we were looking forward to discontinuing the paralytic. Looking around the room at all of the monitors, wires attached to her head, sensor on her forehead…I was struck by an idea: I told Jessica that there was a machine called a neural adaptor that could be connected to one of the outputs and interpret her brainwaves. That interpretation would show on the screen as a digital replica of what she was dreaming. Basically, we could watch her dreams. There was only one of these neural adaptors in the hospital and we would have to ask the nurse if we could use it. She said she did not believe me but I could tell she was partially convinced. When I started to tell Brenda about it, Jess jumped in, "I thought you were joking! That's real?"

"Absolutely," I told her. "It's the latest technology." I clarified that there were many limitations. It was only black and white with no sound and most of the time it only displayed snow, but here and there we would get a glimpse of a horse running, a delicious steak, or whatever she was thinking about.

She was in. As she started to get excited about it, we talked about all of her facial expressions and whether or not her frowning faces were tied to some kind of tough guy fighting dream. As I talked it up, I said how cool it would be to speak to her and watch to see if we could change the content of her dreams. She agreed.

As we came back from lunch, I approached her nurse and told

her that Jessica had a question. Then I turned to Jessica and said she should ask about the neural adaptor. I casually turned my back putting my gown on slowly as I tried with every ounce of my being not to laugh.

"Can we get the machine so we can see Rebecca's dreams?" Jess inquired.

The nurse was confused and after a pause asked, "What do you mean, like an EKG?"

"No," Jess was very clear. "I want to watch her dreams. Can you bring in THAT machine?" By this point, my whole body was shaking because I was trying so hard not to laugh. I was facing away from them but they saw me anyway.

"Arghhhh…RAYMOND!" She scolded as she came over to hit me. "I knew you were lying about that!" She totally didn't know. We both laughed as we went back into the room, though I was probably laughing a little harder.

Bec was doing a little better. I had just nailed a sweet practical joke. Things were not good but they were better than yesterday. For the first time, she hit a milestone and everything worked according to plan. She remained healthy enough to be weaned off the paralytic and bring her a small bit closer to our world. It wasn't great, but it was pretty good.

We continued to joke about things we saw and experienced in the room. One day, Jessica texted me a picture of Kermit the Frog and joked that it was the face Bec made when she was being suctioned. It got me thinking about the other faces she was making. Then, I got it! It was Robert De Niro. She would make this frowning expression all of the time. We started calling her Bobby. Bobby was hard and he took guff from no one! He would stop you in your tracks if you looked at him wrong and he sure as hell wasn't going to let some disease get him. He was tough as nails.

With my friend Norm flying out for the weekend, I looked forward to having another dude in the house. Toward the beginning of his visit, I confided in him: Brenda was getting to be too much. Knowing that Bec and I might both be out of a job soon, it was even more of an irritation that she had not chipped in for groceries. She would help by exclusively doing Rebecca's laundry but would leave it in the washer so when I finally had a minute, I couldn't do the guest linens or even my own laundry. I worried about the timing of any potential guests and even postponed a visit from Mike, Melanie, and Stephanie because I knew Brenda did not play well with others. She would constantly make comments suggesting that she had it the hardest because she was the mom. But it was hard for everyone. In addition to the past few tough years, I had been there every day for a month and was not complaining. The two weeks were almost up and I was looking forward to a break.

I understood that some people found it especially hard dealing with a sick loved one. One day when Jess and I were leaving the MICU, some guy stopped us and angrily told us that we could not be there. He said we would have to take some back hallway because his family was dealing with tough news. I could have just walked through and told him it was a public place and he had no right to stop me. I wanted to and it would be an easy way to work out some frustration. Instead I made it clear to him that everybody stepping out of that MICU had a loved one that was in a tough situation. Nobody was on that wing because things were going great.

As I spoke to him, he softened his tone. He told us that his sister came in the day before and was diagnosed with a terminal condition. I told him I would be willing to walk around but he had to show us the route. By the time we got to the elevator his tone had changed from angry to apologetic. These situations are even more challenging for those who are caught unaware or have not yet accepted them, but it is important to recognize that nobody has a monopoly on heartache.

In a lot of ways, this was how Brenda was dealing with the situation. In her mind, her pain was worse than everyone else's. This can be maddening for those around you who are also struggling. Whatever the situation, whether sitting with other families in the waiting room outside an ICU or dealing with those you know, you should not try to prove that you are suffering more. In some cases it is clear, while in others it is not. Either way it is a competition that nobody wins.

Lesson 11: **There is nothing to be gained by comparing your pain with the intent to prove you are suffering more than others. You will only demonstrate that you lack empathy.**

There are better ways to relieve tension. For me it had always been exercise, whether it was martial arts, lifting weights, or simply doing cardio. Back in college, Norm and I used to lift together and in the past few years we had done four Tough Mudders. During this visit he convinced me to do a half marathon with him in the spring. My initial thought was that 13.1 miles was longer than ideal but we both knew that it would be good for me to get out there and have to train for something. He suggested we use the race as a fundraising opportunity for Bec's transplant. I wasn't quite there yet but it got me thinking.

The biggest roadblock was training but the reality of the situation was that I did not need to be in the room all day every day. If I could step out for lunch, then I could step out for a quick workout. I had joined an LA Fitness which was only a few miles away so it was doable even for a sunny day runner. Weighing around 225 pounds, I was a great runner…considering. In fighting, those in lower weight classes could earn respect as great pound-for-pound fighters. Why should they be the only ones who get an exclusive distinction that considers their performance with respect to their size? What about me being a great pound-for-pound runner? If you took an average runner then packed 50 pounds on him, would they be able to take me? Probably not…so pound for pound, I was better than average!

Between bills, career sacrifices, all of the visitors, and Rebecca's condition, there was a ton of stress. I looked forward to a little exercise therapy. Getting out of the hospital room would help, though unwinding was still hard.

I could relax in the hospital room better than at home because I was not worried about what was happening with her—I could see it. I could bring my bills there, my iPad, and I even had a recliner. In the background, I knew my career was unraveling, but there was no way I could be at work. I met with representatives from my company several times to develop a solution. Though they did not want to let me go, I had no idea when I would be able to return to the office. We chatted about options but the solution would have to wait.

With the girls in the room, Norm suggested that we take a break and go see a movie. I knew it would only be a moderate distraction but I agreed. I loved movies, even the bad ones, and could get into just about anything (especially action and sci-fi) but not that day. Norm had dragged me to the theater to watch *Interstellar*. I remember following it, then my mind would wander back to Bec and I would get this sinking feeling in my stomach and completely stop caring about whatever was happening on the screen. Nonetheless, it was still a distraction and that had value. It was the same case at home. I would just as soon turn on a show as look at the wall. Shows started to look less like a story and more like a bunch of actors walking around saying lines. I could not get engrossed in anything.

Not surprisingly, what seemed to help this was Bec's improving condition. Since the paralytic was discontinued, she was improving in small increments daily. Bec was on methadone because they wanted to wean her from a potential addiction to some of the heavy sedation. This was all progressing according to plan—Plan Z. She would even open her eyes sometimes though she would just stare off into space and was still not communicating. The doctors told us that it could be two to three weeks before she was actually awake and coherent. At this point, any news that was not bad was good. Brenda's visit was also coming to an end and I was looking forward to having my house to myself again. I knew Brenda had wanted to be there when she opened her eyes. She would position herself right in front of Rebecca's face whenever she opened her eyes so she could be the first person Becca saw. The doctors had explained that we had some time before Bec could actually see anyone but she did not seem to believe them.

I knew leaving would be tough for her but I had no idea what was coming. Out of the blue, Brenda approached me with a plan to extend her stay indefinitely. She was going to call the airline and change her ticket to open ended. Up to this point, my philosophy was to keep an open door policy for my home so that everyone felt welcome but it seemed that her staying would add a challenge and a little drama to anyone else who wanted to come.

She caught me off guard and I did not try to hide my disappointment. I did not want her to stay and I wanted to be clear that her attitude needed to change. All I could think to say in that moment was "If you do, you're going to have to start chipping in for groceries." It felt petty and kind of like I just skimmed the nail with the hammer but at least it was something. She told me that she would and that they were leaving for the grocery store shortly.

I sat in the room, dreading the longer stay. I knew that my mother was coming in a few days and I knew that it was going to be a challenging visit if she saw Brenda making this whole situation about her. I kept trying to think of a way out. With two weeks down, another three would stretch this visit to almost a month and a half. She was becoming that roommate who didn't get along with your friends, and I had little remaining energy to host her. For me, this added stress was making an already tough situation, worse. Since Rebecca did not need her at this point, it was purely for Brenda. She wanted to be there when Bec opened her eyes and flights were expensive, but this was not going to work.

January 25, 2015 text to Brenda: *Instead of doing open ended, it might be best if you stick with the original flight or just extend to thurs. It could be weeks before she's coherent enough to remember seeing you. You could be of more help to her later in her recovery.*

I knew we would need to have a talk and was convinced that there had to be a better way. Brenda wanted to be close by when Rebecca opened her eyes and she did not want to fly back to Idaho and then back here because of the cost. After thinking through some scenarios, an idea came to me. An awesome, brilliant idea...

When I got home that night, the girls had shopped and cooked. After dinner I sat for a chat with Brenda. She reiterated that she did not want to leave because of the cost of a return flight. Smoothly, I rolled out my alternative. I suggested that Brenda return to St. Louis with Jessica. She would be only five hours away by car. I would call her when Bec was awake and she could be back here that same day. By the look on her face, I realized that agreement was not so certain. She shook her head and told me that five hours was too far away.

I knew I could sell it. She had not seen her grandson Cole in several years so I mentioned how nice it would be to see him as well. It would cost her no money for flights. If she wanted to come back before Jessica did, the only cost would be a one day rental car. This was only making her more aggravated and she commented on what her friends would think if she came back before Bec had recovered. This seemed like a nonissue to me, as I wished my problems were so minor that my friends' opinions even made the list.

I told her as nicely as I could that she was welcome back but that five weeks at the house was a long time. She asked me to just tell her if I wanted her to leave. I sat there in disbelief wondering why she was fighting this so hard. As we went back and forth, the St. Louis option proved insufficient but it was her unwillingness to compromise that slowly firmed my resolve. It was a reasonable request but she took a hard line. Her conclusion was that St. Louis was too far so she decided to fly all the way back to Idaho. I knew it would be a point of contention in the long run but it was too much to deal with her attitude on top of everything else. Her ire was worth it for a break from the stress.

After giving Jessica an earful for not standing up for her, she booked her return flight and it was not long before my house was quiet once again. Her parting text suggested that perhaps things between us were not so terribly damaged but I never knew with her. We could only hope for better days.

January 27, 2015 text from Brenda: *Thank you Ray for the stay. Take really good care of my Little Girl and please keep updated. Xo*

January 27, 2015 text to Brenda: *No problem. Will do, travel safe!*

CHAPTER 8

ICU Later

With Brenda gone, I only had to worry about the rest of my problems. I was almost out of vacation, personal time, and sick days. Once again, I sat with my company representatives knowing I had little to no leverage. I considered bluffing that I was ready to return to work if I felt I was getting a raw deal because I knew that nobody wanted a half-distracted person at the helm of an important product line. It was the only card I had to play but it was not necessary. They proposed a very reasonable solution that I signed along with a confidentiality agreement. I cannot share the details but I will say it was more than fair and I was relieved to have one less worry on my plate. I suppose I was relieved and disappointed all at once but the good outweighed the bad.

As the days went on, Bec continued to improve. My mother arrived and she helped me with all of my daily tasks. This included moving Becca's joints, stretching her legs, massaging her hands and feet. She took some time to brush out her hair and we watched her

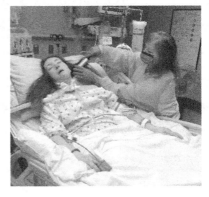

make small incremental improvements.

> **January 24, 2015: Facebook post to the CF page**
>
> *Quick update on how Rebecca is doing...Day 25 on the vent. We had a pretty big scare in the beginning of the week but she's rebounded really well from it. She's still unconscious but they're starting to drop her sedation again. We're just hoping to avoid this cycle of reducing sedation, falling out of sync with the vent, increasing BPs, then increasing the sedation again...*
>
> *Here's to hoping she's having some good dreams in that head of hers.*

In fact, it was such an improvement that they were soon talking about moving her out of the MICU and into a long-term acute care facility (LTAC) called the Daniel Drake Center for Post-Acute Care. Earlier that month, Rachel and I had taken a tour and spoke to the staff there. It was considered the best pulmonary LTAC in the greater Cincinnati area and many of her doctors from UC had rounds there, including Dr. Joseph.

> **January 28, 2015: Facebook post to the CF page**
>
> *Finishing up Rebecca's 29th day unconscious and on the ventilator and we've got something to look forward to...rehab. The doctors have (well) prepared us for the worst, but she's come back strong from a pretty big scare a week ago and I'm convinced that she'll keep making progress, beat the odds, and win this round. I suppose there's no benefit to thinking anything else. Thanks for all of your thoughts and prayers.*

She was becoming more responsive, even though she was still sedated. One day during her blank stares, she was looking at me and I could see her face muscles trembling to do something. They slowly pulled back into the first smile I had seen in a month. I was thrilled! I think my mom and I ate dinner two hours later that night because it was so hard to leave.

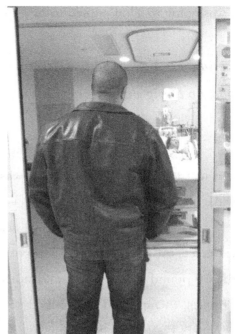

Then, on the thirtieth of the month, I was telling her nurse the story of how we had met seventeen years ago that day. Bec opened her eyes and smiled from ear to ear. Directionally, she was smiling at the sink in the corner of the room but I assumed her aim would only improve and took that as another positive step. Bec was opening her eyes at this point but was not exactly awake.

We were getting very close to being discharged to the LTAC across town. She was still on a ventilator but the edema had started to decrease and she had nearly beaten her most recent pneumonia. Then, seemingly out of nowhere, they were ready to transfer her. They reminded me that there was a good chance she would not make it out of the Drake Center and that it was likely she could be back in the MICU. We were not out of the woods by a longshot but on this day,

I was going to allow myself to be happy.

Lesson 12: You have to celebrate the small victories because they add up to big victories.

Her new room at the Drake Center had a window and a door and just felt more like a home. It was a much better room in which to wake up than the ICU.

When she first awoke, she was weaker than I would have ever expected. All of her muscle atrophy had brought her weight down to the 70-pound range. She could not even reach her face to scratch it. Physical therapy (PT) described it as "not strong enough to resist gravity." This was on a Thursday and her first appointment with PT was the following Monday. I knew from discussions with Dr. Joseph that the only patient with CF that she saw transplanted on a vent was up and walking. Our main goal was strength and I was not about to wait four days. I started working with her in the bed, having her push and pull against my hands with her upper and lower body. I convinced her to do this by promising stretching or massages. This was great deal-making by me because I was providing those regardless, and she was in no state to negotiate with a master like myself!

By the time PT came on Monday, they were surprised at what she could do and Bec enjoyed their reaction. Exceeding expectations was always motivation for her. Regardless of how frequently they came, Bec and I were going to work every day.

I worried about leaving her because she was no longer in the

MICU and nurses had more than two patients. Of course she was on a monitor and had a ventilator that would alarm as well, but by then I had fully transitioned into an overprotective mom. With the trach in place, she was still not able to talk because the air was not passing through her vocal chords. As she became more alert, she would dream a lot and soundlessly talk in her sleep. Once in a while, some air would escape around the cuff (which was a seal between her trach tube and trachea) and it would travel up through her vocal cords. As a result, she would often say one loud word and wake herself up. If only we had a neural adaptor to see what she was dreaming. The Bobby De Niro faces were in full effect however, so I had some idea.

As the sedation worked its way out of her system, she was left a little confused, often forgetful, and extremely hysterical. All of the communication tools were great but Bec was a little delirious and too weak to use some of them. I had an alphabet laid out in a grid on a sheet of paper that we would use when I could not read her lips. She would point to letters, then get frustrated at me for not understanding...W.......H......R.......A. WHRA...? She would shake her head *yes* then I would find out that she wanted a towel or something. Eventually, I learned to ask about the essentials like water or a bedpan first. If that was not it and we had guessed for a while, I'd try to distract her with some of that tapioca pudding with the weird balls in it. Like a senior citizen, she loved that stuff. Meanwhile, I honed my skills at pillow arrangement, EKG sticker application, and fan mastery. The more comfortable she was, the less frustrated she would get in our game of charades.

Cards poured in along with flowers and gifts. We received care packages from family and friends. Meg came out again and among her gifts was a white board. Rachel's family had put together a tool to help us communicate which contained different phrases she could point to.

As she became more alert, she would ask questions, often the same ones every day, starting with, "What happened to me?" I would walk her through everything step by step from the day she was admitted. I felt so much sympathy for her waking up in the hospital, weak and ventilated. The best way I could show her support was through patience. Every day when she asked what happened, I would try to summarize it in about five minutes then wait to see where her questions took the conversation. Sometimes she would pause on new details, but most of the time, she would ask the same things. We would always review the date she was admitted and when she was transferred to the MICU. She would ask what time of night she was transferred and who brought her. I would tell her I did not know who brought her; she would say that she thought it was an RT and that she was so nice. Apparently the RT told her, "You don't have to work this hard." That was comforting to Rebecca. It also made me feel that she was in caring hands at her most vulnerable moment.

I walked her through the events of January then would ask her if she had any other questions. She would say, "No," think for a second, and then proceed to ask me five more. After our discussion, she would look a little depressed and I would tell her that it was a miracle she had survived and that God was looking out for her. She had always told me that she must have an army of angels watching out for her.

I read her the cards from our friends and family to remind her that so many people cared for her. It almost always helped. Her sedation-affected memory was a mixed blessing because I could read her the same cards every time and they were always new to her. I also made sure to tell everyone that she enjoyed them in order to keep them flowing. On a shelf near her bed, I had placed many of the get well mementos she had received. I had a picture of Jesus from my mom, healing stones from her sister, origami from Justin (one of Rachel's sons), and the collection continued to grow. Like her cards, I could show these to her over and over for the first time.

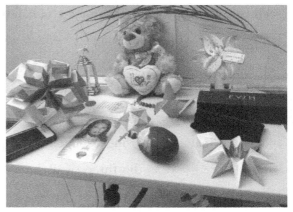

There was a downside to her affected memory. One night at around 3 a.m., I got a call from the Drake Center. It was Rebecca's nurse. She had woken up and did not know where she was and asked for me. I talked to her on the phone and convinced her to take her anxiety medication that also made her sleepy. She agreed and then fell back to sleep. This was the first memory she retained. So after all of the hours I spent in the hospital, the nights I slept there, all of the time she had friends and family near her, the first memory she had in 2015 was waking up confused and afraid in the middle of the night in a strange place. Wonderful.

She continued to get stronger and become more aware. By the time Jessica came back for a visit, Bec was both interactive and entertaining. After passing her swallow test, she could eat real food again. With her hair in a poof on the top of her head, her head wobbled around as she double fisted her milk and ginger ale. Her hands were just as shaky as her head as she took a sip out of one, then the other, then back. Her lips often missed the straw because of her lack of attention and her wobbly movements. The whole time, she seemed to be engrossed in some awful hallmark channel movie that we had turned on for her. Jess and I looked at each other and smiled. She was adorable.

I rolled up some washcloths for her to squeeze to strengthen her hands. A huge grin came across her face as she started shaking them like maracas, missing the point completely. It did not matter. Things were good as the three of us hung out and enjoyed the small victories.

Physical therapy came in to transfer her to a chair but she was too weak to stand on her own so they used a device called a Hoyer Lift and she loved it. She smiled from ear to ear when they lifted her in the air. They settled her in the wheelchair and she started pointing her finger like she was shooting a gun. Trying to read her lips, I came up with, "I'm abata...bataa…" Turns out she was saying, "I'm a badass!" She nodded with confidence. For the first time in the new year, she was having fun! We both agreed, "Yes, Bec, you ARE a badass!"

She made us work to read her lips by talking fast, refusing to rephrase anything, and making up words as she went. We had to decipher, "My glute bone hurts," like that was a thing. She also coined the term "snoozer" and all of these terms quickly entered our daily vocabulary.

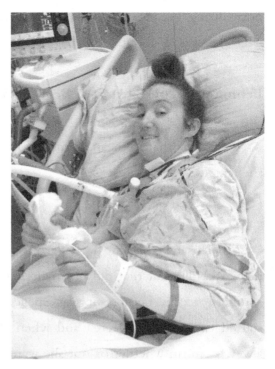

She would often forget that she was no longer at UC hospital and would ask for a cheese Danish thinking that her favorite coffee shop was downstairs. She would slow down on the word cheese so we understood her, "I want a cheeeeeeese Danish…a cheeeeeeese Danish." From then on, whenever we had the opportunity, we would get her a cheeeeeeese Danish.

When I would show her pictures or texts on my phone, she would take it from me and, without fail, would find some way to nearly delete whatever I was showing her, with her shaky fingers and her bad aim. Typing on her iPhone was never her strong suit, however, after six weeks of sedation, atrophy, and delirium she truly sucked at it. When she did try to rejoin the world of texting, autocorrect stepped in to help.

She would awaken in the morning with this urgency for us to arrive, particularly in the beginning. We knew her mental state was normalizing because "anxious with a strong sense of urgency" was what Bec was all about.

February 13, 2015 Text from Becca at 5:46 a.m.: *Can both heart.*

I took that to mean, "Can you both hurry?" Two minutes later, she texted...
Hey Deere ASAP!?????

This text became legendary. I'm pretty sure she meant, "Get here ASAP!!!" but that did not matter. Jessica started saying it with a southern accent because it was spelled like John Deere tractors. I started calling Bec "Deere" and when she asked for things I would always confirm whether or not she wanted it ASAP! Upon our arrival, we found that she was ready to post "*Mmmmmmmmmmmmm CB*" to Facebook. Bec and her shaky fingers were the life of the party.

Meanwhile, her prognosis continued to plague my thoughts. When she asked if she could go home later that week I struggled to answer. I told her that it would probably be two weeks knowing full well that it was unlikely she would ever get to leave. She lay there disappointed while I stood there overwhelmed. She was not only too weak to walk, she was too weak to move herself around in her bed. There was so much work in front of her and I knew that the odds were stacked against her. I wondered if she might go through all of this recovery effort and then pass away anyway. I knew it would not be for nothing but I could not shake the thought.

I needed to rationalize it somehow. I rationalized that every day is a blessing. If Rebecca had passed in January, I would have wanted more time with her. Now I had that, even if we did not know for how long. Every day was an opportunity to talk to her one more time, sharing thoughts and experiences. I decided I would see it as another chance. Regardless of how much time we had before, this time was a gift. I would enjoy every day and would do my best for her—partly so that I would not be left with regret. What was the value of only living for a better tomorrow if tomorrow did not come? It was important to find a way to appreciate today because every day is a blessing.

Lesson 13: Every day may not be a good day, but recognize that it is good to have that day.

We were blessed with these additional days. I did not know how many there would be, but we would make the best of them.

A few days after Jessica arrived, our friends Jimmy and Tracy paid us a visit from Wisconsin. I got the date confused so when they arrived at 2 a.m. I came to the door with a kitchen knife hidden behind my back. Relieved to see a face I recognized, I was able to return the knife to the block without sticking it into anyone first. The next day, they came to the hospital with food and a Wendy's Frosty. Bec was still a little loopy from the coma but she knew what she liked. Her face lit up like a nerd at Comic-Con when she saw the Frosty.

I brought it to her thinking I had a second to get a napkin to cover her trach. I did not. She scooped out an oversized spoonful with her shaky hands and brought that dripping mess in for a landing. I reached out and caught a handful of the stuff in my glove. Acting with lightning precision so the Frosty did not drip all over her breathing tubes I managed to grab a napkin before it truly got out of control. The jury was in and I had a lot of trips to Wendy's in my future.

At the time, I did not think much of a text from Brenda asking me for Rebecca's address. As the weeks passed and she did not send flowers or a card, I figured she had forgotten. However, there was much more going on behind the scenes. Soon after Jessica left, she called me stressed out and concerned. She pleaded with me to drop this thing with Brenda and to try to work it out. I had no idea what she was talking about. She said something about making peace for Rebecca's sake. I told her that we were not in an argument and that she would probably be annoyed for a while but we were fine.

On the other end of the line Jessica was starting to piece something together. Then she told me that we were not fine. Brenda was pissed. This was probably when she realized that this was not a mutual argument and proceeded to explain the situation. Brenda had called Jessica all fired up, with a plan. I had expected Brenda would be annoyed at me for not letting her extend her stay indefinitely, but I had no idea how angry she would become.

Brenda's plan was to get some donations, fix up her fifth-wheel trailer, move it to Cincinnati, and show up at the Drake Center unannounced in March. She was not going to talk to me or let me know her plan. When Jessica suggested that she call me before she came out, Brenda would not have it and accused Jess of taking my side.

She said she was going to show up in person because she wanted to see the look on my face and watch my body language when she walked through the door.

She said that she had "allies." What did that even mean? I had told Brenda she would be welcomed back. She told me to take care of her little girl. We were not always on the same page, but now I was her archenemy? And who were these allies that thought they had a say? It seemed like she wanted to visit her sick daughter out of spite. Though Becca was now awake, Brenda was not going to ask for her feedback either. This move seemed like it was more for Brenda than for Bec. The whole thing was surreal.

Rebecca needed a lung transplant and Brenda was planning to get donations for herself. She justified it by determining that what Bec needed most was her mom—a mom who had, at one point, given her the silent treatment for a year. Brenda probably did not think 'she owed me any communication because she would not need to stay in my house. What she did not understand was that hospital room had essentially become our home, our bedroom really. To show up unannounced and intrude on our time without asking either of us was simply disrespectful.

Jess went on to explain Brenda's opinion on Rebecca's recent hospitalizations. By "making her" go to Colorado and later to Connecticut for Christmas, it was my fault she had become so sick. Not that I expected any compliments, but this was a slap in the face. Aside from the fact that CF is a progressive illness, nobody could make Bec do something she did not want to do. That was at the core of who she was as a person.

Even though she had not lived in the same state as Rebecca for twenty-seven years, Brenda had plenty of theories on Becca's health. After a visit in 2014, when Bec was at one of her sickest points, she had concluded Rebecca was "playing up" her illness for my sympathy. After Becca found out, I had never seen her more insulted. Back then, I reasoned with Bec to give Brenda the benefit of the doubt. I told her that it was probably easier than believing the alternative…that Rebecca was getting sicker. In reality, Becca often tried too hard to tough it out and should have asked for help more frequently.

I sat there alone, imagining what Brenda was saying to her friends as she requested donations to fix her trailer. I could only assume she was telling them about how I was keeping her from her daughter and her trailer was her only way she could be there. I did not really care…but I kind of did. News of this really riled me up, but it would have been way worse if I was caught unaware by a surprise visitor. We needed to have a say in this, but I knew the only one she would listen to——even a little——was Rebecca. I did not want to add any stress or badmouth her mother to her, but I needed for her to have some understanding of what was happening. I had to choose my words carefully.

I decided to just ask Bec if she wanted Brenda to move out. There was no hesitation in her, "No." She wanted her to visit, but was not ready for her to be living nearby and coming in all of the time. Her presence stressed Bec out. That was all I needed to hear. I would suck it up and deal with a long-term stay if Bec really wanted it, but not a "spite stay" and not because Brenda thought she could bully me.

I struggled with how much background to tell Bec. I did not want to detail Brenda's actions in January or how she was railing against me to her family and friends. I certainly did not tell her how excited Brenda was to be able to walk in and surprise me so she could see the look on my face and read my body language. She should have been more excited to walk in and see Rebecca's face and body language, and how she was so much improved from January. I just told her that Brenda did not feel the need to show respect to me as husband and caregiver, because she was mostly focused on her own worries. I told Becca we would work it out but the only thing that mattered was whether *she* wanted Brenda to come out and for how long. Bec wanted her there for a week, so I told her to relax and focus on recovering. I would deal with the rest.

I wanted the best of both worlds, to win the battle without firing a shot. I knew if I confronted her about it, she would make it a standoff and would make it seem like I was keeping her from her daughter. It would be black or white and I would have to either let her do whatever she wanted, or ban her from the hospital. That was a lose-lose scenario.

If she was fundraising, that meant that she was telling a story to motivate people to donate. I suspected that story consisted of me keeping Brenda from her daughter. I also knew that there was no detail about what Rebecca wanted, because she had never asked. I proposed to Bec that we post a little something on Brenda's Facebook page. Together, we wrote a post from Rebecca.

> **February 16, 2015: Facebook post from Rebecca to Brenda's page**
>
> *Hey mom, I was hoping you could come to visit for a week in March. I'm not ready for long term visitors yet but I would love to see you. Maybe we can talk about planning a fundraiser. Please give Ray a call to coordinate.*

This was a fairly tempered response for a situation that Jessica worried could result in "World War 3." I commented underneath the post asking her to call me and mentioning that I had not heard from her in a while. Brenda immediately deleted it from her page. Seeing that, I swiftly reposted it and she deleted it more quickly the second time. All of a sudden, she could not get a hold of us fast enough. She texted me, then texted *and* Facebook messaged Bec. Then she texted me and told me she had Facebook messaged Bec. As I had expected, there was something in that message she *really* did not want her friends to see.

If she had told her friends that I was somehow preventing her from coming out, an invite clearly contradicted that message. If she was fundraising to fix her trailer, then the comment about planning a fundraiser for Rebecca's transplant put things in perspective…this was Becca's addition. To me, the key point was the fact that Bec was not ready for long-term visitors which highlighted that Brenda had not even asked Rebecca what she wanted. I would have been ok with Brenda's plan to move (though not overjoyed) if it was what Rebecca wanted. Brenda had not considered this and she was focused on her own needs.

Lesson 14: Listen to what your loved ones want, even if it is not what you want for them.

She sounded defeated during our call that night and we planned her visit for one week, no conflict, no standoff. Situation averted. Our issues were not resolved, though. Not by a long shot.

CHAPTER 9

Pain and Gain

When Bec first stood up, it took two therapists to help, and after a few seconds on her feet she sat down saying with surprise, "That was hard!" As time went on, she grew stronger. First she was able to stand and then started to walk with a walker. We celebrated each victory with a note on the dry erase board. Her distances increased from a few assisted steps to walking across the room and back.

She was often tired when it was time to walk because she was on a weaning mode (CPAP) on her ventilator. This meant that she would trigger the breaths and get some added pressure support but she would be using her diaphragm and physically working to pull air into her lungs. She could often handle it well when she was sleeping but HATED it when she was awake. The goal was to increase the time in four-hour increments until she was exclusively on weaning mode, and then take it to the next step to a trach mask. We did not make it to the next step.

She could handle an hour or so at a time and it seemed to keep getting worse. Once her respiratory rate crept up into the 40s, the session was stopped. She often did not know when she was on it so whenever she was having difficulty breathing, she would look at me suspiciously and ask if she was being weaned. If I told her she wasn't, she would squint a little in distrust, and then check the vent herself. Her mantra at work was her mantra in the hospital: Trust but verify…with an occasional exclusion of the trust part.

After a few weeks, her lungs were not improving and then they seemed to decline. I was convinced that this was psychological but then they took her for imaging. They found out that one or two lobes of her right lung had partially collapsed. For the pulmonologists, this was the final confirmation that she could not get off of the ventilator with these lungs. They stopped the CPAP altogether. There was nothing new they planned to do about the partial collapse. There was no surgery or re-inflating process. All we could do was increase the frequency of her airway clearance (chest PT and nebulized treatments) with an additional focus on her right side.

The new direction was to focus all of her energy on walking. She also received a new goal, 500 feet in six minutes. This was one of the requirements for the University of Michigan Transplant Center. The goal seemed achievable which made the transplant start to seem like a real possibility. She had beaten the odds in January. Now we needed to build the strength to do that again.

As she increased her distances, she had to deal with the anxiety of using a walking vent. This was a portable ventilator with settings that were different from the one in the room. When it came to the walking vent, she had to breathe differently, it felt different, and her anxiety would often get the better of her. There was an RT that she worked with, Ann, who was the ONLY RT she would work with when walking. Between Ann and Denise (who planned her workouts) we got a routine down with the goal of walking frequently and slowly increasing distances.

If Ann was not there, there was roughly a zero percent chance that Bec would switch to the portable vent and walk. Her increased anxiety always played a role. On days she did not walk, we did "bonus" standing exercises by the bed. Our biggest challenge with getting her workouts in was the amount of time she would sleep…and that woman could SLEEP. We had a small window between snoozers to do any kind of workout. Sleep was important and I did not want to disturb her too much, but sometimes it was a huge impediment to progress. And lack of progress could be a huge impediment to her spirits.

Every night before I left, I would tell her I was proud of her. One night she looked at me and told me, "I believe that you are proud of me, but I'm not proud of myself!" It was hard to hear—well, to lip read. Bec was her own toughest critic. When she was put under in December, she was able to do all of this. Then she woke up in February and could not even reach up to scratch her cheek. She was comparing herself to months past when she should have been looking at the previous week.

I talked her through every improvement she had made, one after the other. She had gone from immobile to standing and walking. She had gone from ICU delirium to comprehension. She was getting physically and mentally stronger every day. I reminded her about how sick she was in January and how she beat the odds. It takes time to bounce back from being so sick and she needed to have patience with herself. I continued to tell her I was proud of her but I needed her to actually believe what I was saying and not just humor me. So like a tenth- grade English student, I had to prove my case with examples. I included specifics of how she improved. I would talk about the number of sets and reps, the frequency of walk breaks, distances, and number of workouts in a day. I would compare these numbers with where she was the previous day or previous week. I felt like a walking encyclopedia of Becca facts but it seemed to work.

I did not want to let her down so I would make it a point to ask her to exercise with me frequently. She did not want to let me down so she would agree to it if at all possible. As a result, she made some solid improvements. She built herself up and would walk longer distances with fewer breaks to rest. Relatively quickly, she built herself up to walking 250 feet and I knew she would reach the goal of 500 feet. She would find the motivation to do what she needed to do, even when she was clearly tired and did not want to move.

I would comment with super funny jokes every time she had a good workout explaining to her therapists that this was no challenge for her. I would suggest that maybe they could get some little hurdles she could jump over or cones that she could weave through. I was determined to make those jokes land so I repeated them daily until everyone recognized the humor.

As time passed, she began to build pride in her own accomplishments and reset her point of comparison to the current year rather than years past. She knew whether she had a good walk. Motivation was critical. Periodically reading her the get well cards and reviewing the gifts we had received helped but I had one more ace up my sleeve. I took the cats to the vet who examined them and signed an approval form so that they could come into the Drake Center. With her cats approved, I could bring one or both of them in whenever she was having a rough day or needed a pick-me-up.

Lesson 15: Look for those things that bring joy and make them a part of your routine.

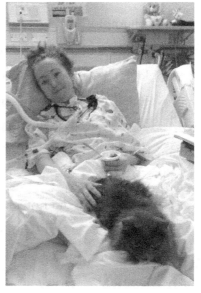

It turned out that Paul was a great guest, though Priscilla was not. After a few instances of crawling on the floor to pull Priscilla out from under a shelf, I decided that pictures of her would have to suffice.

Fortunately, Becca's delirium had passed by this point and it was nice to have her back. I still had some items to check off the list and both required a notary. I got a power of attorney so I could have an actual conversation with the insurance company that managed her disability checks. Next, I helped her complete her will to protect myself—just in case. I watched her sign these documents with handwriting that, for the first time in our lives, was messier than mine. She still had severe muscle atrophy and I sympathized, but I took the opportunity to point this out to her...for motivational purposes, of course.

CHAPTER 10

Rant and Rally

"MY BUTT! Lord, my butt. Ohh lord…lord my BUTT, MY BUTT!!!" we heard over and over one evening. I was so proud of my father for not laughing out loud immediately. All three of us showed amazing restraint sitting there in the hospital room. Almost a full minute passed before it kicked in and we each let out our inner seventh grader.

Becca had a neighbor who we would hear from now and again, a little old lady we'll call Ms. Carla. Ms. Carla was not happy about being there and she made it clear to everyone, loudly. She would often argue with the nurse's aides and then ask visitors to help her. It was not her fault; I believe she may have had some kind of dementia. It was all part of the sights and sounds of hospital life. Ms. Carla reminded us that the struggle can be tragic and funny at the same time. Though it's important to be aware of people's feelings, these situations often held some humor. I could simultaneously feel sympathy for Ms. Carla (and her butt) while also laughing at what she was saying. There is nothing wrong with smiling at the world around us.

Lesson 16: If you have the opportunity, laugh.

Aside from Ms. Carla's butt commentary, it was often a challenge to find reasons to laugh. Rebecca's prognosis had not changed but she did not understand the gravity of her situation. She knew that she could not get off the ventilator without a transplant but she was not aware of her immensely unfavorable odds at getting listed. I felt I should not fully confide in her and risk adding to her anxiety and worries.

It was no surprise that I found myself talking much more to my mother and Rachel. I also found myself speaking to Jessica more frequently. Initially it was updates and medical plans but it quickly moved to how to deal with everything, then basically everything else under the sun. Sometimes our conversations would shift to more spiritual discussions. Jessica's beliefs seemed unique to me and she explained how her belief in nature also drove her beliefs on healing. In January, she had brought some healing stones and crystals to keep by Becca's bed. One type of stone was fashioned into a bracelet which we placed on her wrist during much of her time in the MICU. Even though Jess believed that Jesus lived, she did not recognize him as any kind of savior. As she continued to explain her beliefs, she added a surprising twist: these were Becca's beliefs as well.

It first hit me as odd. I knew my wife would not just change everything she believed without mentioning a word of it to me, so it did not make any sense. My wife's beliefs were similar to mine. We had discussed faith and religion many times. Those conversations would usually conclude with a comment on how we *should* start going to church. But nothing like this had ever come up and if she felt this way, she would have definitely shared it. Faith was not something that we struggled to discuss and Becca knew that I felt everyone has the right to believe or not believe whatever they wish. However, this should not be kept a secret from your spouse. Jessica tried to comfort me explaining that this was not a big deal to Bec and that Bec believed as Jessica did, but did not actively practice this form of spirituality. It was a change that happened a few years ago but she worried more about other things in her life. Jessica told me that maybe it was an oversight because Becca had so much on her mind that was more important to her. Her health was declining, her job was consuming her time, we had dealt with a stressful move, and her weight was decreasing as quickly as her energy level. She seemed to really nail Rebecca's stressors, but Bec and I had always made time to talk...

As she explained this, I thought back to the past year or two and reflected on how Rebecca had grown more distant. It sometimes felt like she was mulling over several serious conversations to have in the future. I always wrote it off as stress. I now realized that this could be a part of it. As Jess spoke with confidence about *their* beliefs, I began to consider that Bec may have changed but did not trust me enough, or have the energy to bring me along. The excuses that Jess supplied only made it worse.

This all made me angry at Bec, not for her beliefs, but for not sharing this fundamental change with me. If I did not know this, how well could I know her? Here I was, sacrificing my career, dealing with family drama, enduring the heartbreak that comes with a drawn- out illness, and she did not trust me with her beliefs? It suddenly felt like we did have real problems, but what could I do? This was not the time to address anything. Hell, she was still making sense of her new reality. Despite our issues, two facts remained: she needed my support and this was not the right time. If she did not want to share her changing beliefs, I was not going to force it. In a perfect world, it would be great to talk things through so I could get all of my sensitive feelings worked out, but that was not my reality. The sacrifice I needed to make was to shut up and focus on supporting her because that was what she needed the most. It might take some strength and self-discipline, but if she could work as hard as she was working, I could deal with this for a bit longer.

March arrived and the issue continued to weigh on my thoughts. One night I sat in my recliner in the corner of the family room with a glass of scotch, just thinking. I thought about this version of Rebecca that Jessica had described. I wondered if Brenda would try her stunt anyway and move out, getting in the way of plans for private time and chances to reconnect with my wife. I thought about the anger Brenda held and what she was saying about me. I thought about Becca's slim chances for survival and the road ahead. I could not stop my brain from circling around these topics over and again, and it came to a point that I had to write them down. I had never kept a journal but that night I understood its value.

March 1, 2015 Rant on my iPad

It has been 61 days that Rebecca has been on a ventilator and she is still working hard. The days are focused on PT and how much work we can get in before she's had enough or falls asleep. She hasn't given herself enough credit for the improvements she's made and (as always) discredits my encouragement as bias or ignorance. So we try to stay focused on the 'next goal'.

I walk the line between saying all of the things I thought of when she was unconscious...and keeping quiet so her nights in the hospital don't become a dreaded time to overthink. You cannot underestimate a positive attitude but you also cannot silence your own needs completely in the hopes that illusion of positivity for someone else will have more value than your own struggles.

So as the tempered words and crafted sentences escape, I know I'm simultaneously imparting too heavy of a burden while selling my own needs short. It is compromise tied to a ticking clock so I know I'll never have the time to figure the plan out just right, but if I don't start executing it soon...it will fall to dust in my hands.

So I sit here at an epic crossroad with an urgency to say everything while knowing that I could regret so much of it. All the while, she has a mindset that was barely influenced by the life changing experience that she has put me through.

I make sacrifices that I can't tell her about. I've been defamed by those close to her, but is it better to not say anything? I've learned of parts of her that she would not share with me even though I shared everything with her. I have plans for the future but they may be compromised by sugarcoating the present.

In the end I could spend way too much time trying to live up to my ideals and developing a perfect approach to only be dragged down into the muck and cheapening all of the good I feel I have done. So off to bed I'll race because I've got to sleep too little, wake up too late, and race back into a situation where my best contribution would be to shut up and smile while spouting unaccepted cheers into the ear of someone I think I know.

It was one of my lowest points. Aside from the fact that the scotch might have amplified the melodrama a bit, it was a pretty accurate description of my state of mind. I had been unable to clear my head of those thoughts as I tried to sort out my feelings. Resolution would have to wait because I needed to put on a happy face and go in the next day ready to lift up and motivate.

I also hoped that one day, the opportunity would be right for me to talk openly with Rebecca about these issues. If that day ever came, I absolutely needed to capture the weight of the situation. I think that part of the reason I was replaying it in my head was that I wanted to remember it well enough to convey it.

Lesson 17: *Writing down your thoughts can provide the impetus you need to move on.*

I firmly believe that God does not give us anything we cannot handle. Therefore, if I had all of this on my shoulders, this must mean that I was that strong. By this point I believed it and knew what I had to do: keep moving forward.

Days had become much more demanding which was a nice distraction. My role increased from an occasional application of lotion and some range of motion movements, to a full schedule of activities. Rebecca did not like the hospital food so I always brought alternatives. I would end each night by mixing her favorite yogurt with a variety of fresh fruits and coconut oil then putting it in snack size containers to bring the next day. Added confidence in her condition meant I did not expect a late night ICU phone call. This allowed for a new step in the process called tequila.

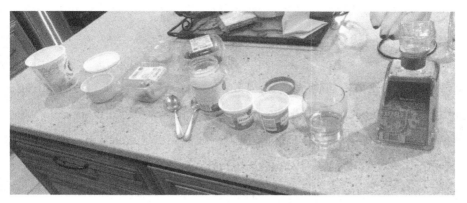

Per her specific requirements, I would bring Kozy Shack tapioca pudding, Boar's Head cold cuts, and whole milk in a small cooler. Dry goods would go in my reusable grocery bag along with bills and other paperwork. This particular bag, from one of Rachel's care packages, advertised some colon cleanse product. It had, "Shit Happens" on the side and seemed quite appropriate.

When I arrived, I would usually have to do some pillow adjustment while she told me she did not sleep well. I would help her to the commode and got pretty good at managing her lines. At some point, we would transfer her to the wheelchair but with her increased strength, we no longer needed the Hoyer Lift. Lotion and massages continued daily to make the day more pleasant. We targeted one stretching session and two workouts each day. I would shave her legs and cut her nails when she needed it. I became a master of brushing out her hair and putting it up. She never admitted that it looked amazing because she must have been jealous of how good a stylist I had become in so short a time.

My lip reading skills improved a bit and she finally slowed down, so we could actually communicate. When her food would come, it would typically sit for several hours because she was on her own schedule. Once reheated, I would rearrange her table, place a napkin over her trach, then talk the food up as if it was appealing. Preparing and grabbing snacks and drinks were in the job description as well. We collected an entire closet full of food. If nothing suited her fancy, I would head to Wendy's for a baked potato or some chili…and ALWAYS a Frosty thanks to Jimmy and Tracy. I felt like I was popping up and doing something every twenty minutes—probably because I was popping up and doing something every twenty minutes.

I would try to be there for rounds but the timing was a little less predictable than in the MICU. There would often be one issue or another they were trying to resolve, usually having to do with her gastrointestinal (GI) tract or her heart rate. I would get the daily phone extensions and call the nurses and RTs whenever needed. They taught me how to suction her which I would do if necessary but they preferred that I waited for them to do it because they needed to log it…and probably also because it was their job.

In the evening, she did not want me to leave until she was transferred back into her bed from her wheelchair. On the way, we would stop off at the commode then I would get the toothbrush and water ready. I would lay out her bedside table with everything she might need during the night. I would keep the water close, lay out a snack if she got hungry and included Creon (her digestive enzymes) to take with the snack. She might need juice if her blood sugar went low and her glucometer to test it. The iPhone had to be a safe distance from the water and seemed safer on top of the napkins. Every night I presented her Kindle to her as a great alternative to insomnia, but she would just give me a Robert De Niro nod as if to say, "Fogetaboudit," often immediately after I made the suggestion. Before I could get over to my jacket, she would have identified a few last things to keep me there. Tasks like brushing her hair or stretching her out were common. This was an ideal time to get her to do any of her exercises that we may have missed during the day.

Finally I would tell her I really had to go, citing the time (usually 8 or 9 p.m.) and that I had to eat dinner. If she wanted me to stay later, I would tell her to expect a later arrival in the morning. Unless there was a valid reason, getting a full night's sleep was critical. I noticed that I needed this both physically and emotionally as the weeks went on especially because there were no weekends and no vacations.

Lesson 18: A full night's sleep, whenever possible, must be a priority.

This was my job all day, every day: making her comfortable, physically and emotionally. I tried not to complain because I was grateful for the fact that she was there requiring this of me. And how could I complain? Rebecca was in a hospital bed practically 24/7, could not speak, and could not physically do most things on her own, like breathe. In combination with her type-A personality, I knew this was torture for her. So compared to some people I had it tough, but compared to Rebecca, I had it easy.

Fortunately, Rebecca was focused on the here and now. She spoke much more about her immediate comfort than she did about her long-term prospects related to transplant. In part, it was because we had a plan, but that was not the biggest reason. This was her personality. She saw things tactically and focused on how to achieve clear goals that were directly in front of her. If she had my personality, and worried more about the long term, I think it would have been harder for her to stay motivated. We were both lucky that she was who she was.

March continued with more improvements for Bec, slow but steady. Her edema had gone away and she fully looked like Rebecca again. She was mentally alert as well, even though she struggled a bit with her memory. Increased physical strength allowed her to move around in the bed and better reach the items on her bedside table. When we spoke about her improvements she would usually respond with, "Getting there." That was the closest she came to giving herself a compliment.

Gaining that confidence in her condition helped me step out of the room and kick off the training for my half marathon. Though we were on the other side of the city, there was another LA Fitness nearby and the Drake Center was set on a large campus with a one-mile path marked around the buildings. I would wait for her afternoon snoozer then change for my workout. Running was good therapy and I reminded myself that if she could get out there and walk on a ventilator, I could run whatever distance was in my plan that day. At times it was a little boring but perhaps that was due to my slower speed (but respectable momentum). Lifting was more enjoyable but not the priority, so I only justified a few sessions per week. Working out was the one thing I would do for myself every day, physically and mentally.

During many runs, my mind would drift to Rebecca's condition, visitor timing, insurance issues, and finances mostly. Slowly, these worries would fade and most times I would return to her room exhausted yet rejuvenated. There was good and bad that came with it as I would build up an appetite, then have to resist all of the junk food everyone had sent to Rebecca. More importantly, I had found something that I could do if I had the chance. I spent way too much time watching her sleep to argue that I did not have the time. During challenging times, people will offer you free excuses. They will say that it is understandable to skip workouts. Sure it is. I missed many workouts waiting for a CT scan or a bronch. But the bottom line is that the benefit of exercise outweighs the justification of a good excuse.

Lesson 19: Make the time to maintain an exercise routine.

As unimportant as it might seem at times, it is an investment in your own mental and physical well-being. It is a release for when too much bad news hits at once. It is a break to help provide perspective. As L'Oreal says, "You're worth it."

CHAPTER 11

The Spreadsheet Champion

We had always expected that Rebecca would one day require a transplant. What we did not expect was the nature of the illness preceding it and the impact of its duration. The plan was to buy our home based off of my salary only. This way when she could no longer work, we would be fine. Insurance would cover most of the medical bills, our savings could cover other related costs, and my salary would continue. Though we expected to have two more years, we had saved a respectable amount. Since I needed to stay with Bec and we were stretching into the third month, I would ultimately not have a salary. That meant that at some point, the mortgage would be coming out of the savings and it would only be a matter of time before that savings ran out.

I did what any self-respecting engineer would do, I developed a spreadsheet. Week by week I walked through different scenarios. How long could we continue at home? If she was listed, what would be our living expenses near the transplant hospital? What was the impact of a long wait for lungs? I attempted to answer all of these questions but the answers were rarely encouraging. I saw no way around having to fundraise. I had done so for the CF Foundation in the past but it was different to do so for our medical bills. It felt a little too much like failure. Every scenario had a different date when we ran out of money but there was always a date. If that date came before her transplant and I was unable to cover her insurance premiums, I would have failed her. If we somehow worked that out, I was pretty sure I would be on the road to bankruptcy. That was not an option, so the decision was clear. I would have to swallow my pride.

After some research, we decided to go with Children's Organ Transplant Association (COTA). Donations would go to COTA and then we would fill out a form for qualifying expenses and receive a check, which was categorized as a grant, to cover these costs. They could provide tax receipts to the donors and even an additional $2,500 grant if we reached the $25,000 fundraising mark. When I inserted *those* assumptions into my spreadsheet, it improved my projections quite a bit. Everything I had researched told me that COTA was a great organization. Their people were easy to work with and Rachel volunteered to take the lead as the community coordinator. Between work and family, she still managed to find time to be the point person for the campaign, taking a huge burden off of my shoulders.

As fundraising ramped up, a message showed up on the page from one of Brenda's friends believing she was the admin. She inquired whether it would be better to send the money to Brenda or to COTA. I told her who I was and clarified that only the COTA donations could be used to help with Rebecca's medical bills. After her donation, I sent her a thank you to which she responded and clarified that it was "for B and her family." She wished a quick recovery to "her (Brenda's) baby girl" adding, "They're still our babies no matter how old they are. No need to reply, just give Brenda a hug of support from me."

It was sort of odd that she avoided offering me any consolation or even referring to her as my wife. And the "No need to reply"? What did she think I was going to say? I suddenly had strangers sending me words of wisdom from across the country. Her note confirmed my assumption of what Brenda had been telling her friends about me. I had to remind myself that it was inconsequential.

The timing of Brenda's visit was planned to coincide with Jessica's next trip. I knew she would not drop the idea to move out here. I told Rebecca that if that was what she wanted, I would be fine with it, but that I did not want her to feel pressured by Brenda. Bec still wanted a visit and nothing more. Her mom could be hard to refuse. Anxious about a potential discussion, Bec found just the right words. Then, she forgot those words. I helped her remember them...and she forgot them again. We wrote them in her phone, and then she fell asleep. I knew if Rebecca agreed to it, Brenda would feel she had a mandate to be there so I had expected her to force the discussion. To my surprise, she did not.

I started to relax after that first day. Letting the girls have their mornings together allowed me to get some long-delayed things done around the house. Jessica's son, Cole was visiting as well, so I even got a little help with the patio set. The whole visit was going off without a hitch.

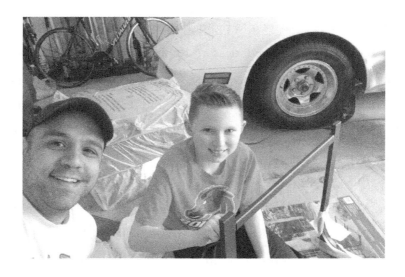

Back in the hospital room, Jessica took care of whatever Becca needed…hair brushing, feet rubbing, commode retrieving, and all so I could truly take a morning off. I had hoped Brenda would get into the action as well and fulfill her Becca fix, but Facebook and her phone were more appealing. I had expected after all of the drama and plans to move out that she would have doted on Becca nonstop. That was not the case.

Brenda was notably absent during Rebecca's first walk of the visit. Disappointed, Bec asked why she had not come to watch. With her increasing distances, she was finally starting to take pride in her walks. Though it was a large enough space, Brenda's reasoning was that she did not want to make it too crowded. I suspected that she did not want to risk losing her comfy recliner. In either case, wasn't this why she was there—to provide support?

She did want to buy Becca a snack, so after a swing and a miss with a gluten-filled pretzel, I suggested the Wendy's Frosty. I had not bought one in a few days and figured that would make everyone happy. Upon receiving her prized dessert Rebecca announced, "This is the second Frosty I've had this year." What!?! I must have bought her more than fifteen Frosties since Jimmy and Tracy left a month earlier and she had forgotten all of them? Of course I could not get mad at her memory...her crappy, crappy, memory.

On one of the last nights of the visit, I treated everyone to dinner. We shared some Becca stories and enjoyed a few margaritas. Jessica told a story about how I had stood up for Rebecca with one of her nurses who had a bit of an attitude and was not being as careful as she should have been. In her way of trying to bring people together, she was clearly trying to show Brenda how I was advocating well for her daughter.

Unimpressed, Brenda explained how she would have done much more. She would have fired that nurse because she does not accept any nonsense. She then went on to retell the story about when Bec was a child and how Brenda stood up to the doctors who had trouble diagnosing her. As we walked out of restaurant, Cole and Jessica thanked me for dinner while Brenda was oddly silent. That was when I realized, she saw me as her competition. Maybe it was because she wished for a better relationship with Bec, maybe it was something else. Whatever the case, it seemed to ring true.

After they headed home, we shifted our focus to transplant options. While Becca was getting stronger, I was learning a great deal about lung transplant programs. I had received a list of programs covered by our insurance—thirty-seven of them. I started to research each one to select and prioritize our application process.

The first of the selection criteria was the quality of the program. Surprisingly, every site touted an amazing reputation when describing their center. I found a *U.S. News & World Report* rating various pulmonology programs. I also learned that we wanted hospitals that completed at least twenty transplants per year so that the staff maintained adequate transplant experience.

I reviewed the United Network for Organ Sharing (UNOS) website and was able to find some great statistics. One-year and five-year survival rates were great points of comparison. We wanted approximately 80 percent and 50 percent respectively, for these timeframes but that would not tell the whole story. If a program accepted tougher cases, I would expect the scores to be slightly lower than more exclusive programs.

The next category was their exclusivity. Was it likely that their acceptance criteria would exclude Rebecca from consideration? My information in this category was sparse because most hospitals did not have well defined criteria listed on their websites. They would tout some of their tougher cases and I was looking for anything about transplantation from a ventilator.

I considered location knowing that this would have a big impact on our finances. We could potentially be spending a lot of time there and would also require several trips back and forth. Location near friends, family, or our home would gain additional consideration.

The final category was the expected wait. Time was of the essence and I wanted to find a way to understand this. UNOS provides information on the number of people listed and transplanted in the previous year. This is broken out by organ and even by blood type. This was not the best way to look at it because the allocation of donor lungs is by region and score. The country is divided into twelve regions and a lung allocation score (LAS) is used to assign each patient a relative priority in that region. I did not know how many people each region included nor did I have their scores. Each LAS is assigned upon listing so I also had no idea what Rebecca's score might be.

All I could do was gather the information and sort through it. The most logical way was to do so in a spreadsheet…an amazing Ray Poole Spreadsheet that had hyperlinks and a comment column for added details. Perhaps it would be filtered and each category would be ranked on a scale of one to five then tallied, giving an overall score to each potential facility. Yes, Rebecca needed a spreadsheet and I was going to develop one.

We quickly prioritized our list and sent the top three to Karen, the social worker for the CF clinic in Cincinnati. Barnes Jewish Hospital in St. Louis was first and Jessica and Trey had offered to let me stay there if that worked out. Duke University Medical Center was second and was near our friend Meg. University of Wisconsin Hospital and Clinics was third and was more like a safety school. We figured that was a definite *yes* because they had cared for her for a decade.

Like movie doctors always say, "We did everything that we could; all we can do now is wait and hope." I was actually beginning to feel more hopeful. As I researched fundraising organizations and transplant hospitals, I had to think through everything from possible transplant timing to housing options. Even with my spreadsheet mastery, there were a lot of variables. In January we were told to hope for the best and plan for the worst. I found that we needed to plan for the worst and for the best…and then plan some more.

Lesson 20: Plan for the worst, plan for the best, and plan for everything in between.

CHAPTER 12

Unimportant Trach Noises...
Unless They Matter

One issue inevitably gave way to the next. As her stomach issues subsided, breathing issues began to present themselves. There seemed to be two major problems. The first issue was with the cuff. This was a balloon-like component that encircled the trach. When inflated, it would seal the space between the trach tube and her trachea. This ensured that the air being pushed into her airways went down into her lungs and not up and out of her mouth. Occasionally air would escape past the cuff and make a loud sound. This startled Becca every time and added to her anxiety. The only way to stop the sound was to increase the pressure in the cuff. Unfortunately, higher cuff pressures increased the outward pressure on her trachea and over time, could stretch it out and weaken it.

Rebecca would always ask her RTs to increase the pressure because she hated the air leaks with a passion. The RTs would describe her trach as "positional" because slight movements would cause it to make noise. To me, it looked like it was moving too much with respect

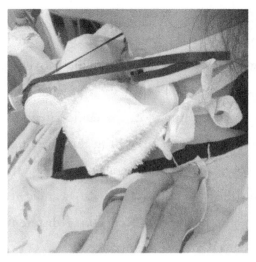

to her neck so I secured a rolled up washcloth to prevent it from sagging downward. It seemed to work reasonably well.

The second problem was much more frightening. Something would go wrong and she would be unable to breathe. We would also hear some cuff noises but in this situation her breathing would become notably labored. RTs could not figure out what was wrong. They looked at the volume of air she was receiving and everything looked like it was fine. As it went on, her vent pressure measurements would start jumping around and her O_2 sats would begin to drop. Often she had to be bagged to bring her levels back up. It was scary for everyone and nobody could figure it out. After it had happened a few times, one RT tried to tell me that her volumes were okay and I snapped back at him, "She clearly doesn't look okay!" Between the sedative (Ativan) they gave her for her anxiety and the exhaustion from the experience itself, several hours of sleep would always follow. It could sometimes wipe her out for an entire day, often causing her to miss her critical PT appointments. This was causing both immediate and long-term harm.

I wanted an explanation of what could cause the pressures to change like that. Figuring that out seemed to be the key to resolving the issue but nobody could explain what was happening. They suggested we change her trach to see if that would fix things. Bec was not sure what she wanted to do. She feared a trach change but wanted to be compliant. She was following my lead and after talking it over, I told the doctors we declined. I wanted a good explanation of what they would do differently and if they could think of a specific situation where this could explain her symptoms. They brought in the attending physician who proposed one theory, that it could be a hole in the cuff though that did not fully explain the symptoms. They also wanted to try an adjustable trach which might position the cuff in a different location in her trachea. That convinced me and I convinced Bec.

Minutes later they were prepped and starting. Bec was visibly nervous. I had to stand clear so I sat across the room hoping she could stay calm. Her nurse was a short, round, older lady who stretched herself all the way across the bed to reach up and hold her hand during the procedure. Her holding Rebecca's hand helped us both feel better.

The fellow started the procedure then I could see something was wrong as they became more anxious and I heard terms like erosion, granulation, and tracheomalacia. Issues continued as the attending took over and still couldn't place it. Finally, they brought in a completely different trach and they decided to use that. We had hoped for a simple fix, but had discovered more problems. Erosion described tissue that was worn away from the inside of her trachea. Granulation was damaged tissue. Tracheomalacia was a condition in which the tracheal support cartilage lost rigidity, possibly leading to tracheal collapse. High cuff and vent pressures were taking their toll on Becca's trachea. We had no idea how long it would hold up or how long it needed to; we needed to talk to an ear, nose, and throat (ENT) specialist.

A few hours later, I noticed that the trach was sticking out of her neck pretty far. Her RT seemed to think it was ok but the next thing you know, she could not breathe and they had to bag her again. Watching her panicking and afraid never got easier. I suggested marking the position in some way. That did not work and neither did the trach change, it was a rough day.

On the ride home, I got a call from Pete. This was not uncommon and he would make a point that he was calling to see how I was doing. Though at the time I had trouble separating Bec's medical condition and my own spirits, it still felt like another person on the team had my back. His work made it challenging for him to return, but he supported the costs of Jessica's numerous visits and that was the best way that he could help.

I had told everyone that if they wanted more detail than the Facebook updates, just call. Though I often wished for better news, I gave them the whole truth. That night, all I had was a treatment plan and a bunch of potential options. Her treatment consisted of steroid drops and an upper limit for the cuff pressures. The ENT could propose a more aggressive fix like surgery, to cut out the granulation or insert a stent. Temporary measures, as I interpreted them. This increased the urgency of getting the transplant. How long could her trachea hold up?

We were still trying to process this news when we heard back from Barnes Jewish Hospital. This was our number one choice. It was a good hospital and it was located right near her sister in St. Louis. The answer was no. They would not transplant her; they would not even evaluate her for transplant. Five years earlier, she had cultured the harmful *B. cepacia* bacteria. Antibiotics had been able to knock it out almost immediately, but doctors at Barnes were afraid that it could re-emerge after the transplant. They rejected her immediately upon seeing this. Jessica was convinced that they took tough cases, so if that was true, the odds were less in our favor for the next hospital. Karen called me with the news and I had time to process it and decide how to present it to Rebecca.

It was not meant to be and we were lucky enough not to have wasted our time or money transferring to St. Louis for evaluation. We would much prefer to be turned down sight unseen than waste precious time on something that would not work out. It was time to focus on the next hospitals on the list and reasons why we thought they would accept us. We had truly dodged a bullet. I thought about how terrible it would have been if we had bankrupted ourselves flying out there back in January, and then got turned down. By the time I told Rebecca about it, I had rationalized all of this and did my best to explain the good and bad of the situation. It still sucked.

Meanwhile, Rachel and her family had arrived for Easter and my dad was already visiting. We had a full house and we were going to enjoy the holiday. The plan was for me to go to the Drake Center in the morning, go home for an early dinner, and then bring her meal back to her room along with the whole family.

I arrived in her room to find Becca sleeping like a baby. She remained out for the next hour. This was typical. Shortly after she awoke, Rebecca could not breathe. As with every other time, thoughts raced through my head that this could be it. That they would try but not resolve it, and I would lose Bec right there in front of me. I hit the "O_2 breaths button" (which increases the oxygen to 100 percent) and just as I headed into the hallway, her RT was coming to the door. The RT came in and held the trach in different positions until Bec said it was a little better. She deflated the cuff, repositioned it, then re-inflated it and it worked. This was enough to tire Rebecca out and it was snoozer time again.

As I imagined the worst case, I began to picture that sometime later the doctor would explain what happened and it would turn out to be some risk that I did not know existed. My imagination would have to stop there because I was not going to mourn someone who was still with us. I suddenly felt a strong need to take advantage of this time and have a serious conversation. The Easter holiday had pushed the question of her beliefs to the forefront of my mind. It also provided the right backdrop for a conversation about it. I wanted to talk to her that morning.

When she woke up, I wished her happy Easter and we started to talk. I asked her if she believed in Jesus. She said *yes*. I made it clear that I was fine with whatever she believed; I just wanted her to be honest with me. At this point I half-believed that she was lying to me. She looked at me like I had two heads. When I explained what her sister had told me, she was very clear, "No, that's what Jessica believes; it's not what I believe." I asked her one or two times in different ways and she came back with the same answer. She had not changed her beliefs. She was adamant and I was quietly relieved. She had not been hiding a whole side of herself from me. This was the Rebecca that I knew.

As we continued, I wondered why Jessica would tell me that. She always had good intentions and had been helpful throughout this whole journey. I knew she was only telling me what she thought was the truth. I wanted to text her, or call her to tell her what Rebecca had said. Bec had not kept this side of herself from me — it did not exist. I knew Jess would think Rebecca was just trying to make me happy but I could prove that was not the case.

I thought that maybe it would be better if Becca told her but she seemed to have little interest in doing so. I sat there thinking and slowly came to another realization. The motivation to tell Jessica was for my benefit, not for Rebecca's. What difference did it make if Jessica had the wrong idea of what Bec believed? Either she would not believe me or she might feel the same way I had after our first conversation on the subject. Neither answer was of any benefit to Bec or to Jessica. Her motives had always been pure and this was a miscommunication. I was happy, she was happy, why try to fix it? So I let it go.

Lesson 21: Be aware that when you get something off your chest it could end up on someone else's shoulders. Sometimes there is little value in setting the record straight.

I left the room feeling better than I had felt in a while. It was a beautiful day but the night was even better. We got to the hospital with her dinner and some gluten-free desserts. Oddly, Rebecca had not only received her dinner tray, but she had eaten the whole thing. For the first time in three weeks she ate a meal on time and it happened to be when she was waiting for us to bring Easter dinner from home…great. I should have told Kindra (her favorite nurse) to stop in and remind her that dinner was coming, but I somehow let it slip. I could not really get annoyed at her filling what little space she had in her stomach with hospital food because her memory was still spotty. She had just forgotten about the dinner from home, and that was ok.

Regardless of this, the night was fantastic. She loved her Easter basket and gifts but the highlight of the night was my niece Gabrielle playing her guitar and singing songs. She played for over an hour and it was so nice to be having fun in the room with Rebecca. I was not worried about getting home for anything. All that we needed was right there in the room. On the ride to the airport in the morning, my dad described it as bitter sweet. There was no better explanation.

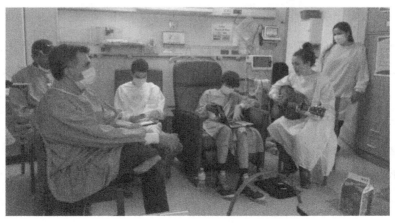

Left to right: Ray (Sr.), Michael, Justin, Jeremy, Gabrielle, Rachel

The next morning, I got in early and found Rebecca had already experienced another incident with her trach. These were happening multiple times a day now and after finding out about her trachea damage the previous Friday, I was anxious to get the ENT appointment scheduled. PT was now being canceled proactively in order to avoid making the issue worse so I sat there thinking about what exercises we could do in the bed.

As she lay there sleeping and recovering from her morning I became more and more concerned. It seemed like there were very few breaths without the sound of air leaking out. It was not her biggest problem, but it was a source of anxiety for us both. We learned that she could avoid it by taking shallower breaths but that was not really a solution. After a second incident occurred, we were getting continual updates from the RT. Discussions with the pulmonologist and the ENT were ongoing and they were nearing a plan.

The pulmonologist came in to propose we move her back to the MICU for better access to the ENTs. The other benefit was that we could expect a faster response because each nurse only had two patients instead of six. The transport presented a whole new set of concerns since incidents would sometimes occur just from Becca sitting forward. Now we were going to put her on a mobile bed, change her vent, transport her across town with a team unfamiliar with her, change her vent again, and provide her with a whole new staff. Adding to this, that day Rebecca had a new nurse who started out by putting her enzymes down her feeding tube and clogging it. Then, after bringing them in late, she spilled some of Bec's anti-anxiety meds just before the transport team got there. As the nurse was getting a towel Bec was fuming, "That's it! She's done! Tell her she's done!"

Afterward she got so upset and she started to tear up. I knew it was awful to have no voice in addition to this medical nightmare she was living. Crying, she just kept saying, "They don't listen to me!" It broke my heart. She was overwhelmed and I wished there was more that I could do. The last thing I wanted was for Rebecca to deal with more anxiety but it was almost unavoidable at this point. She had not received her anti-anxiety meds until the transport team was already there and they took a while to work. Plus, she only got a fraction of the dose. With all of this going on I decided to ride in the medical transport with her and take a taxi back to get my car later. By this point it was already 6:30 p.m. and we weren't on the road yet so I figured it would be a long night. I figured right.

The transport went surprisingly smoothly and soon she was in her new room. Getting set up in a new hospital takes patience and now it was time for my anxiety to begin. Nobody was wearing gowns. I told the nurse that she should be in reverse isolation and she told me she had not seen the order and did not know what the doctors would decide. I told her, "I know what the doctors will decide and you're just going to need to listen to me because I'm this close to kicking everyone out of the room until this is resolved!" Perhaps I did not say that verbatim. Maybe it was more like, "She should be in isolation because that is standard practice with CF patients and it has been strictly enforced since January." But I said it sternly because I was getting fired up. I also considered resuming my former role as a bouncer until they resolved it. After telling the nurse twice, a doctor walked in and we got it resolved.

Transitions were never easy. Though it was another UC hospital facility, they still needed to re-setup all of Bec's orders and medications. This meant ensuring the tube feeds would start that night, discussing the insulin plan, and discussing how they should administer her Creon. I worried that a quick break from the room could mean a mistake not caught in advance.

Her breathing was labored so much that even sleeping exhausted her. The problem was that this vent was not the same model as the one at the Drake Center and had different settings. We called respiratory to adjust the settings multiple times but never fully resolved it. I could not leave her there alone that night so I got my car and returned for another restful night in the ICU. I somehow hooked myself up with another one of those recliners that won't stay fully reclined unless you hold it there—fantastic design.

They scoped her twice that night and once the next day. Each time, the verdict was the same, the trach was in a good spot, there was nothing they could do about the tracheomalacia, and they didn't think her tracheal damage was severe enough to cause the problems she was having.

She had an incident during the third procedure and they watched through the scope as she brought up a mucus plug which blocked her airway. I saw her mouth the much too familiar "I can't breathe." I hated to see her in that state again but I hoped that they would determine a clear diagnosis with a simple fix, like in a good episode of *House*.

Unfortunately, with the diagnosis of mucus plug, our plan was not new or exciting. It was more of the same, airway clearance. It was further confirmation that we needed to get new lungs before these ones crapped out. The fact that three ENTs came to the same conclusion was both good and bad news. Surgery was not needed but we still had no solution. I did not want to go back to the Drake Center to more of the same. The only other explanation we received for the situations when she could not breathe was panic. At first it seemed like a panic attack could not cause this issue until I thought back to the PICC line removal incident in our bathroom ten years earlier when she passed out with her eyes open. Note: I will never do that again.

As I started to match up symptoms, I started to come around to the theory. The sound of the cuff leaking stressed and startled her — what if she panicked? Initially, she would still be getting her appropriate volumes and the RTs would not be able to find anything wrong. If she started hyperventilating, that would cause the pressures to start jumping around as her breathing accelerated. Hyperventilation would lead to dropping oxygen levels which always followed. This also explained the brief losses of memory she experienced because that had also happened during the PICC line removal. Note: I will not even consider doing that again.

The focus had to shift to keeping her calm and giving her tools to avoid panicking. This was a plan we could act upon, and I started feeling better about our return to the Drake Center.

CHAPTER 13

Tenacious B. vs. B. Cepacia

Meanwhile, I still had a half marathon to train for and had now missed two days of training. Luckily, the versed they gave her for the last scoping procedure knocked Bec out and provided me with a couple of hours to get home, run 5 miles, shower, and get back. Unfortunately, it was drizzling when I got home so there was no possible way I could run under those conditions. In life, when Plan A doesn't work out, it's necessary to have a Plan B. Mine involved watching TV, eating some cookies, and finishing them off with a muffin. I was now fully carb loaded and ready to sit in the recliner. I should have saved my comfort food for a little later, because I was about to need it.

Karen called and it was more bad news. We did not get accepted into the University of Wisconsin transplant program. This was a tough one to take because Bec had been a patient there for ten years. They typically did not accept people on vents but had been willing to consider Rebecca. However, added risk from previous cultures of *B. cepacia*, liver disease, low BMI, and her "borderline" kidneys complicated the decision. Ultimately, the previous *B. cepacia* culture was the reason.

This hit us like a ton of bricks, not only because it was our contingency, but we had now been turned down twice in a row. As I was hearing this news and looking at Rebecca sleeping, I could not help looking at her incredibly skinny arms and legs. At least before there was always some level of edema, so even if it was just water weight, she did not look this small. When she stood up earlier that day she was clearly weaker than she had been a week earlier and it might be another three days before they could walk with her again. She was 87 pounds at this point and yet again, my mind went back to whether or not she would survive. Would we apply and be rejected from program after program, wasting time while her health continued to decline? Now I worried how long her trachea could hold up and how much time we had before her next pneumonia or exacerbation hit.

We sat with Karen and Dr. Joseph to discuss our new plan, the shotgun approach. We applied to her next few top choices: Duke, Michigan, New York-Presbyterian/Columbia University Medical Center, and University of Pittsburgh Medical Center (UPMC). Duke was her number one choice before getting sick. They did 130 transplants a year with a great one-year survival rate (greater than 90 percent) though the five-year rate was in the forties. Michigan had good survival rates and decent volumes, though they had twice as many people listed than they transplanted in the previous year. New York-Presbyterian was geographically close to my family in Connecticut and had survival rates similar to Duke's. I had hoped this was because they both took tough cases.

We had not considered UPMC because of some of the stats I had pulled off the UNOS website. Apparently, I had grabbed info from the wrong hospital or something. I tried again, and learned that they did as many transplants as St. Louis and Wisconsin combined, about 100 per year. I already knew from the CF page that they took tougher cases and it was only four and a half hours from home.

I left that conversation excited about the shotgun approach and hopeful that we would be hearing something positive in the next couple of weeks. Anxiety about the situation was rising a bit but I could not let Becca see that. As we left the hospital to return to the Drake Center, I was consumed with thoughts of her pending reviews by these transplant programs. We were re-settling into her old room and it did bring me some comfort when Rebecca said she was glad to be back and that she liked it here at rehab. It was the only home she remembered from that year. Many of the staff stopped in to say hello and Sue (an RT) even brought her a cheery decoration. It felt like home.

With the edema gone, Bec finally realized how much weight she had lost. She kept saying she needed to gain weight, and asked for an increase in her tube feed because she knew that some hospitals had a minimum BMI requirement. I asked her how much she weighed and she said 103 pounds. I was glad she thought that because she would have been more discouraged if she knew she was in the eighties.

But the number I was watching closely was her heart rate. There was a fine line between understanding her trends and overreacting to a blip; however, she was ten minutes into a snoozer and it was 127 beats per minute (bpm). She was talking so much in her sleep that her eyes were opening. I quietly sang "The Beccalicious

Song" hoping that would calm her. I softly put my head to hers and my hand on her arm, just trying to calm her without waking her. Eventually her heart rate dropped to 105 bpm, but even that was higher than her past norm.

After staying elevated for a few days, her tachycardia (elevated heart rate) began to concern her doctors. They put a rule into effect that she could not do any PT if it was over 120 bpm. Unfortunately, this was where it averaged, so we began missing more opportunities to walk. We tried to time her naps so she would wake up just before PT and it would still be low from the snoozer. It worked about half of the time.

Bec was still having episodes where she could not breathe. Now we were trying to understand whether it was panic-driven hyperventilation or mucus plugs that triggered anxiety. It could be some combination of the two, but I suppose it did not really matter because the fix was the same: slow, controlled breathing. It was much easier said than done, and not very feasible if panic had started. The concern that there would be more incidents made it harder to leave the hospital, or even leave her room.

As her spirits began to drop, I knew the timing of Scott's visit could not have been better. He was a calming presence for her and I was glad he could see her in a better state than in January. It was also nice that she would have company when I stepped out to run.

One day I got back from a run and she was on the commode with the curtain drawn. Over the sound of the vent, I could hear a tapping. I knew she wanted her privacy but I peered around the corner anyway because I don't listen so good. She was tapping on things around her to call out for help because her trach was stretched taught and it was pulling. I preferred to arrange things in the room because I was so used to it but since I was running, somebody else had set her up. I gave her some slack while we worked on breathing consistently and slowly, but I could see the panic in her eyes. It was like watching an accident that you could see coming but were powerless to stop. As her breathing rate increased, the sounds of the ventilator and her noisy trach seemed to get louder. Luckily, we got her back in her chair quickly because the panic was setting in. All I could do was talk to her and hold her hand as she became less and less aware of me. I asked her to look at me and concentrate on my voice, but I could see in her eyes that she was starting to lose control. As she looked at me less and less, her eyes rolled back in her head and her mouth pulled into a grimace. I knew she would be okay but I kept thinking about her father, who had entered during the chaos, watching his little girl. We had to end these incidents or they could sabotage her physical therapy, improvement, and her overall state of mind.

After a tough incident like this, it became clear how good it was for her to have her dad there. She would look over now and then and smile at him, just happy to see him. He would often walk over and kiss her hand. He did not say a lot but you could feel the love they had for each other. As he was by her bedside that night, I could see her saying something to him and starting to tear up. I stepped out and gave them their time but it was bittersweet to see this strong woman in a moment of vulnerability and sharing it with her dad.

That mood continued into the next day. As we spoke about transplant center options and I explained the plan and potential timing. I could see that she was concerned but it surprised me when she held out a thin hand for each of us to hold and cried again, this time with even more tears. I could not help but tear up as we all sat there together, concerned with what the future would bring. I had to remind myself that in January, I would have given anything to have a moment like this—with Rebecca awake and us facing this together. The calm presence and emotional recharge of having her dad visit was so good for her. It seemed to ease her state of mind as we moved into the next week.

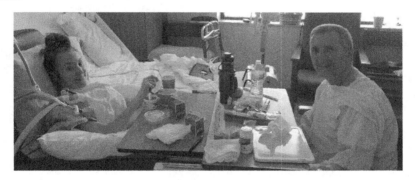

Her energy levels started to improve which resulted in a couple of great PT sessions. The spring weather was here so I asked if they could bring her outside. She was thrilled when they agreed! We got outside and she just lit up. She smiled as she closed her eyes and they wheeled her through the courtyard. For the first time that year she felt the wind against her face and the sun on her skin. We sat there enjoying an experience that had been so easy to take for granted in the past. On the ride back, she stopped for a cheeeeeeese Danish. It was a good day.

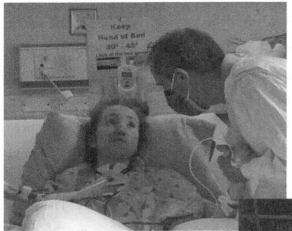

As Scott left, Jessica tagged in again, which was great because it was a huge help in maintaining Becca's spirits (and she was also able to knock down my backlog of dirty dishes). The goal was to keep Becca relaxed and optimistic.

However, we arrived to find a very anxious, uncomfortable lady. Her heart rate was elevated for the third straight day and this time it had reached 140 bpm even at rest. We could tell she was particularly tired and even if she had the energy, they would not let her walk. To top it off, the pulmonologist stopped in to give an update on transplant centers and we had more bad news. Duke and Michigan had now declined to list her and she was down to Pittsburgh.

She took the news in stride and commented that she felt good about the remaining options. It was undeniable that we all felt the impact of it. It hung in the air during that dreary, anxious day that held no answers. Soon, the pulmonologist fellow provided another theory on her tachycardia. After seeing her hemoglobin blood concentration, he thought it might be a hydration issue. After getting some fluids, her heart rate started to drop and went from 120 down to 97 bpm that morning. We hoped we had it nailed.

Her attending pulmonologist, Dr. Elsira Pina, came in to see her. She had seen Rebecca after the Denver trip that past October, in the ICU in January, and several times at the Drake Center. It was clear that she was contemplating something and she paused before speaking. "You're tenacious! You are more tenacious than any sputum in your lungs. I think about you on tough days and know that if you can do what you're doing, I can get through whatever minor thing I'm dealing with in my life." She got a little teary and so did Bec.

It was true; she was an inspiration. It made me so happy that they could see the fighter in Bec. They could see what I saw in her. Dr. Pina spoke about how she often thought about Rebecca. She commented about her support and looked at the two of us standing by her side. I knew without a doubt that we had the right doctors and the right care and we were where we were supposed to be at that time in our journey. As Rebecca teared up, I put my hand on her leg while her sister grabbed her hand. It was a touching moment in a tough time.

Rebecca had earned herself a new nickname: Tenacious B. Fortunately for her, it had too many syllables to use it ALL the time and abbreviating it TB was unfortunately inappropriate. But I *would* use it.

The tachycardia had not fully resolved and they decided to do a

CT scan. They were concerned with a pulmonary embolism. Rebecca's echocardiogram showed that her heart failure had worsened since October and that we might need to bring her back to the MICU for a longer stay this time.

As we continued to get turned down by transplant centers, I recognized that this could only hurt matters. Beyond that, of course, was the concern that this signified a decline in her condition. The physician did mention a combination heart-lung transplant. But this was worrisome because it was challenging enough to qualify for new lungs alone. I only recently learned that the combination transplant existed and had no idea what it entailed. This was just one opinion and her pulmonologists might think this was ridiculous, so we tried not to get too worked up over it but it was the weekend and we would not find out for days.

When we did find out, there was good and bad, as usual. First off, her heart was worse, but not that much worse. She also did not have a pulmonary embolism. They believed that the tachycardia was a progression of her CF and there was not much they could do about it. I was still not sure that this was the sole cause but there were no more theories on the table.

We waited until Bec fell asleep and decided to find a lunch place with an outdoor patio. Beer and wings out on a patio in the spring is hard to beat. As we finished up, a text came in from Bec saying that panic attacks suck. She must have been going through hell while we were just sitting outside enjoying the sun. I could not stop the rush of guilt I felt. Maybe we could have helped if we were there. At a minimum, we could have provided a bit of moral support. Stepping out, even for a short time, always came with worry. I was running when she had experienced her last panic attack. Even being immediately outside the building, I could not help her.

Guilt continued to rear its ugly head. I felt guilty for not arriving earlier in the morning and guilty when I had to leave her at night. If anything happened while I was out I would feel selfish. I would not have needed to go out to lunch if we had made sandwiches. I would not need to run for hours if I bailed on the half marathon. I could come in earlier if I just planned to nap in the recliner. No matter how much I did, I felt I could always do more. I had great support from friends and family, but the responsibility was mine. It boiled down to the question: how much was enough?

What I learned was that there was no correct answer. If I slept there every night and did not leave for a run, sure I could gain a few more hours, but I would wear myself out in no time. I did not want to be tired or grumpy with her. I needed to be positive in order to help keep her spirits up. I also needed to keep myself out of the loony bin. For me, over one hundred days had passed with no day off and more bad news than good. If I did nothing for myself this whole time, I am sure I would have broken down by this point. I had to look at this as a marathon, not a sprint.

Instead of asking how much I could do, I focused on what it was that she needed. I knew what she needed by her expression, her reaction to my planned runs, her anxiety level, and by her medical status. If she needed me I would be there but she did not need me

24/7. I would not always make the right call because I could not predict the future. By the same logic, I should not blame myself after the fact for something I could not have known. The only way I could blame myself for not being there during a panic attack was if she told me in advance that she planned to panic at 2:05 p.m. Being there all of the time was impossible. If that was the minimum expectation I had for myself, then my best would never be enough.

Lesson 22: There is no way to do everything for someone else all of the time. Try to recognize when and how you are needed the most.

This lesson became more important as the weeks dragged into months. I also had to learn to trust her caregivers. Well, trust but verify.

Her heart rate remained high and remained a major concern. She also had a high white blood cell count signaling infection and she had cultured another bug, MRSA. This was a type of staph infection that was new for her. Additionally, she was diagnosed with tree-in-bud opacity. One might think they had finally run out of real names for Rebecca's ailments and had reached the point of making shit up. But the tree in bud opacity was a condition that was diagnosed during imaging and related to issues with the small airways. The physician explained that it was something that people with CF often demonstrated.

The only good news that we received was that imaging had

shown that her right middle and lower lobes had mostly re-inflated from the partial collapse. I was not sure what this meant in the big picture, but a win was a win.

His larger concern was MRSA. I asked him if it was one of the worst bugs and he said unequivocally, "Yes." The infectious disease doctors could change her antibiotic but we needed to act quickly and get her started on vancomycin.

I did what I always tried *not* to do—I googled it. The full name was methicillin-resistant *Staphylococcus aureus*. I saw descriptions that included the term "superbug." I sat there reading, looking at my wife who had been sleeping in the recliner all day. My "what if" scenarios started to creep back in again. Could we knock it out with Rebecca's already compromised health? How could this affect her potential transplant listing?

I noticed her cheeks were sunken in quite a bit that day. Despite our efforts, her weight had been continually dropping and her last weight was 84 pounds. Looking at her skinny legs clearly bothered her. Standing up one day she reached back to feel her butt. She looked so let down. She did not say anything but I knew she was thinking about how skinny she had become and how her weight could affect her overall health and chances for transplant.

When she awoke, she commented to me that she had been trying to eat well—as if she needed to make an excuse. I told her I was so proud of her because I knew how hard that was for her. I counted up the calories of her Boost shake, pudding, whole milk, and beef tips she had for lunch—about 800 calories. Added to her other meals, the snacks, and the tube feed at night, and she was consuming over 3,000 calories a day. The problem is that people with CF are not absorbing it all and what they do absorb gets used up quickly in the fight to breathe.

I told her about the MRSA diagnosis and she was upset. She said she had never cultured this bug in any other hospital stay but I had to remind her that she had never been in the hospital for this long and in such a compromised condition. I saw the sides of her mouth droop slightly, as they often did when she was struggling to stay awake. I was overcome by an awful feeling. I gave her a long hug and could not help but tear up. I wished I could have hid it from her but all I could think about was this MRSA and what damage it could cause. But Becca said it was common, and in true Becca fashion, she played it off as more of an annoyance than anything else. I figured the truth must lie somewhere between her interpretation and the physician's.

Over time, the worry and anxiety attacks were starting to increasingly affect her as I could see her acting more depressed. She had little interest in food and when the poor food services lady came for her order, Bec lifted the cover from her current meal to reveal a less than appealing reheated burger patty and gave her the "really?" look. Instead of a two -minute order process, it lasted fifteen, as we walked through every alternative they had. In the end it would not matter because she would just eat cold cuts and tapioca pudding from our cooler anyway. Meanwhile, I was trying to shove some ham down her throat before PT came around. I made it incredibly appealing by wrapping it with lettuce and tomato from her burger but I couldn't convince her to take a bite quickly enough. The next thing you know, PT walks in the room and the window was officially closed.

We could all see that she was just physically and emotionally exhausted. It was too early for her next dose of Ativan and she had no food in the tank. With her eyes closed, she mouthed, "I don't want to do anything." I told her that it might feel good just to stand and stretch her legs knowing she could stay on her vent. She begrudgingly agreed but started complaining that she couldn't breathe. A few minutes of standing and we were done. She asked me to brush her hair, she got her Ativan dose, and then passed out. As I brushed her hair out, I could see the unrolled ham and lettuce from across the room. Lunch fail.

I did not mind the brushing. I was glad that she liked it so much and that it relaxed her. I had done it frequently since the MICU and considered myself an expert. Of course when she'd ask me to do it she would tell me to start at the ends and work my way up. This was insulting to a man of my experience and clearly she forgot how good I was between each session. I had to put it up on the top of her head in a little poof when I was done. It had to be the top because if it touched the pillow, it tangled. I learned to twist the elastic one to two more times than my instincts told me. I was quite good.

The thing I hated about it was the amount of hair that would come out in the brush. There were handfuls even when it was not tangled. I had no point of comparison for how much was a lot, but there was a lot. It could have been hair that I would feel breaking when I brushed it or the result of her head rubbing on the pillow, but what I did not want to think was that it was from her body letting it go because of her deteriorating health. I could see portions of scalp through her once thick hair and knew that she was unaware of how it looked. I dreaded the day she would find out but maybe things would be going better by then and it would already be growing back. Ultimately, I knew brushing her hair relaxed her like nothing else, so I would do it whenever she asked for it. It was my job.

CHAPTER 14

Transplant Evaluation, a Good Thing

My phone rang with an out-of-state number but my hands were wet and I was kind of a screener anyway. I would grace them with a return call if it was compelling enough. It was Pittsburgh, UPMC—the last and best option on our list! Crap!

I called the lady back immediately and got her voicemail. Double crap! It was twenty entire minutes before she called me back. Rebecca had made it past their initial evaluation, and they wanted to evaluate her onsite! After being rejected five times in a row, we had a real chance. I was told that approval from Aetna could take two to three weeks but I took it upon myself to grease the skids. I waited a day then called to make sure Aetna was prepared to provide a quick answer. They told me they had not yet received the request from the hospital. I was bounced around to a few different people while we sorted out who was supposed to do what.

After getting some instructions for UPMC to follow, I called them (now as an insurance expert). We got things moving along but they brought up that Becca's insurance terminated in about a week and a half. Rebecca's job had been dragging their feet for weeks in sending the COBRA information and now it was urgent. There was no way I could let that delay her approval and potentially her transplant. I told them that I would provide an answer quickly but that it was my expectation that the approval process would continue to move forward. They assured me that it would. About five calls and a few hours later, I got the COBRA process started.

In the midst of all of this, I got a call from Brenda. This was the second time she had called me since January, so I figured it couldn't be good. First she asked if Pittsburgh had accepted Rebecca or if there were more tests. I was surprised that she did not know this from my texts but I explained how they wanted to evaluate her themselves and that this was standard practice for most hospitals. Brenda was annoyed because she was not aware of this and said that it would be easier if the doctors would just come to Rebecca. I suppose it would be.

I explained that this was good news because the hospitals do not want to waste their time with an evaluation that they think will fail. Becca had made it further with UPMC than with any of the other hospitals. It was exasperating having to explain the best news I had received all year to someone who acted like it was terrible. She explained to me that it was very frustrating for her not to know if Bec would be accepted. I refrained from saying that I dealt with my frustrations by being thankful that she might have a chance to live.

She went on to tell me that she was planning a fundraiser in Idaho. I said that was great and I asked that she touch base with Rachel on the requirements for COTA. Brenda told me she was NOT going through COTA. She would do it her way. I explained that Rebecca signed an agreement with COTA and she could not receive funds

LESSONS FROM A CF CORNERMAN

through any other source or her contract would be voided and we'd lose access to the $13,000 we had raised so far in Rebecca's name. I explained that the requirements were not that challenging but promotions must be worded in a particular way and payments had to go to COTA directly. She told me that most folks at the Elks lodge where she worked were not online. I told her they did not need to be and continued to ask her to learn the requirements before saying they were unreasonable. I asked that she just connect with Rachel who would help with whatever she needed. Brenda wanted to do it on her terms and continued searching for alternatives. When I held my ground, she got frustrated and told me that if she could not do it her way, she would just raise money so that she could come out and stay with Rebecca. She said it as a threat which pissed me off because Becca had already told her that she was not ready for long-term visitors. I told her we are raising money for a transplant that her daughter needs to survive and that it did Becca no good for Brenda to raise money for her own travel. Without pause, she went back to talking about other ways that we could avoid using COTA.

I calmed myself down and told Brenda I would talk to Bec and see what she wanted. It was the best tool I had because Brenda was not about to listen to me. I knew that Rebecca did not want her planning a long-term stay and she definitely did not want her taking money that could otherwise help with her transplant. I talked to Bec and no surprise, she wanted to follow the contract she had signed. She was upset and disappointed that her mom was again talking about fundraising for herself so I texted Brenda.

April 23, 2015 Text to Brenda: *Bec wants you to follow the requirements she agreed to with COTA and not risk voiding her contract. The requirements are simple so it shouldn't be much of an inconvenience. Rachel's number is...*
Bec did say she'd be upset and disappointed if you fundraised for your own travel when she is in so much more need for the funds. Let us know what you decide.

She responded quickly.

Text from Brenda: *Really??? The fundraising for travel expenses would have been a cover and a way to get around Cota. Everyone knows that I am fundraising for her. So do the people here.*

Not only was she backpedaling but she was trying to make it appear that it was insulting for me to even think she would do that. But she had just said that to me, directly, and as a threat.

Text to Brenda: *That was how it came across and I know that was your plan before. In either case, Bec wants to follow her agreement.*

The next day I asked Bec to text her asking the same thing. It annoyed me to no end that I needed to bother Bec with "Brenda Management" with the little energy she had. But Brenda did not respect me or my role so sometimes I just needed the boss to put her foot down. It was a lot of aggravation for nothing because it never went any further than that. Brenda never called Rachel and she never planned a fundraiser for Bec. I supposed it was her way or nothing.

Another night of little sleep and her new muscle relaxer for her back spasms made her exhausted. She had about five Creon and four other pills to take that morning and I remember it just taking forever. She would swallow one pill, and then look down while breathing heavily. I asked if she was having trouble breathing but got no response. I waited a few seconds and offered the next pill and she would get mad at me for rushing her then look down again. It took over ten minutes to take all of the pills. The entire day was like this with everything from eating to using the commode. She would see me sitting in my chair and motion for me to come over. I could read her lips just fine from my comfy chair but I would get up, walk over, and she would never tell me, often getting distracted or falling asleep before she could get it out.

In her wheelchair, she spent almost two hours getting situated. I would recline her, she would ask to be reclined more, start coughing, and then ask to sit up. She could not get comfortable, but she was giving me almost no feedback on what she wanted. I tried to be patient but I had a ton of things to do. Along with follow-ups on COBRA with her former company, UPMC, and Aetna, I had received another hospital bill for charges that should have been covered. I still needed to send fundraising emails out for the race that was now next weekend. In fact, I needed to get a training run in before I ate.

I started to get frustrated when she called me over to help her get to the commode but was not ready to get up and did not answer me when I asked if she wanted a few minutes. Then she started talking to the RT who was not looking at her so he could not read her lips. I asked if I could communicate something for her and she snapped at me to "just wait a second!"

I said, "Fine let me know when you need something." I sat back down and started browsing Facebook in defiance.

There was something wrong but what was it? I started to prepare her for the night. I got her table situated with her things, and as she saw me organizing her tray, and she looked up at me so concerned and helpless. "I don't want you to leave," she told me. I was not going anywhere.

Her difficulty focusing got worse the next day. At one point she had to pee so I prepped the commode and told her to stand when she was ready. She looked like she was trying to say something but could not find the words. All of a sudden I looked down and she had gone while sitting there. Something was very wrong. I wondered if it was due to her new anxiety medication. The psychiatrist had come in during a panic attack, so maybe it caused her to overprescribe. There were also new antibiotics and a muscle relaxer. The nurse's opinion was that she was not acting abnormal but she was "off." I asked her to hold the anxiety medication and muscle relaxer.

When the doctor arrived it was like I had brought my car to the mechanic and it stopped making the sound. Bec was surprisingly coherent and interacted with no problems. Fortunately, he trusted my explanation and it turned out that the muscle relaxer was the cause. Way simpler than I expected! Over the course of the day she became more and more aware. By the time I left that night, she was back to normal. Another situation resolved.

During the frustration of those two days, I thought about the entire process of supporting someone else. On day one, it is so easy to hop out of your seat and do whatever you can for the smallest request of a loved one. Day 101 is a little bit tougher (even on a non-muscle-relaxer day). Of course empathy is a strong driving force, but sometimes I would see the same urgency in her request to clean up the bedside table. I learned that for Rebecca (and her type-A personality) it came down to control. Seemingly overnight, she could no longer do anything for herself which meant if she was going to avoid feeling helpless and frustrated, she needed some measure of control. I had to recognize that it was not that the table was urgently messy. It was about her need to control her environment. That often tempered my response from, "Do you really need that right now?" to "Should I postpone my phone call for ten minutes?"

And like a greeter at Walmart, when you have accepted the job and have shown up—smile. Nobody wants to feel like a burden. Often the sacrifices we make are not that epic and sometimes you have to close your laptop and mute your phone because you're going to spend the next twenty-five minutes moving pudding and water bottles around. The *Deadpool* trailer will still be there on the internet when you get back.

The instance with her muscle relaxer seemed to mess with her (already spotty) memory. We talked all morning going through what had happened again. As I hashed through all of it with her I could only imagine what it must feel like. She felt the doctors could have avoided giving her the trach. I had to tell her again how very sick she was and how the doctors expected that she only had days to live. She still did not have a concept of how close she was to death.

It sucked explaining all of this again. Again I had to convince her that she should look at this situation as a good thing. She was there because she survived and the only alternative was not being there at all. She was still alive because she had overcome an incredibly tough battle and she still had more fight left in her. As I gave her the pep talk, I started to bring my own mood back up. She was a fighter and at that moment she was so much healthier than she was a few months ago.

Throughout this experience, I noticed that trying to bring others up often made me feel better. I had learned in January not to mourn someone who was alive. I would not be shocked if the worst case happened, so why not also look at the best case scenario as a probability? The true risk was being miserable, not surprised.

I found myself see-sawing as my mind naturally wandered back to the worst case scenario. I would reject that, try not to mourn, then I would try to refocus on what I was looking forward to. The positive swing came more quickly when I was trying to lift up Rebecca's spirits or helping someone other than myself. The key was to focus on actual facts. We could talk about what she had overcome, her current treatment goal, and her future transplantation options. Explaining why a particular concern was not so terrible helped me believe it.

This also seemed to apply to the sympathy situation. I could justifiably sit around moaning, "Woe is me." People would easily sympathize with me, feel terrible, and say they could not even understand what I was going through. It was nice to hear, but generally did not make me feel any better. It was the equivalent of them putting their hand on my back and rubbing it in slow circular motions saying, "There, there." It's sweet, but a little useless.

When I told people what she had been through and how she

kept fighting they would be impressed. If we spoke about what she was currently dealing with, I would focus on the plan. Instead of getting a ton of sympathy in return, I would get encouragement: sure she will get strong enough; the body is an amazing machine. She sounds like a fighter. You guys have such a great attitude. These responses did more to bring me up and I would often leave encouraged.

People look for cues from you. If they hear you saying how nothing will work out, they will comfort you, which almost confirms your worst fears. They do not know if things will get better or if you want to hear that. Give them some direction, and by doing so, help yourself stay positive.

Lesson 23: People will respond to what you provide. If you want them to help you stay positive, show them how.

The day started great with Rebecca eating three bowls of cereal and looking alert. It started to go downhill quickly, as she could not get comfortable or decide where she wanted to sit. Therapy was at 2 p.m. that day so I had asked the nurse to bring in her Seroquel (an antipsychotic) and blood pressure medicine a half hour before it started so it would start working in time.

Ann was out so I had called another RT and asked her to help by managing the portable vent. Right before PT came in, her heart rate increased from 117 to 120 bpm which was just out of range to allow the therapy. We stood there and watched to see if it would come down but it didn't. She sat and fidgeted, complaining that she could not get comfortable while we watched her heart rate creep up to 121...122...123 bpm...then float around in that area, frustratingly close to the acceptable range required for physical therapy. It never happened.

She asked for more Ativan but needed to wait for the doctor because not enough time had passed since her last dose. In the meantime, we turned down the lights, I kneeled in front of her holding her hands, and we started her new relaxation app. This was a progressive muscle relaxation technique, during which she would tense and relax different muscles as the voice from the app guided her through the process. I could see her concern in the form of the many wrinkles that were bunching between her eyebrows. We arrived at the portion of the exercise where she was told to stretch her mouth open as wide as she could. With such a worried expression, she opened her mouth in a long silent roar, showing all of her teeth. As a mature adult, there was no reason to believe I had a huge grin on my face under the mask. Then out of nowhere, Bec opened her eyes, looked at me, and said "I know you're laughing!"

"This is my favorite part of the exercise," I told her. Then she went back to panicking and I went back to kneeling uncomfortably on the floor...totally not laughing at her. When the faces unfortunately stopped and the snoozer began, my thoughts went back to the events of the day. With some thought, they had actually reinforced the notion that everything happens for a reason. We were so frustrated that her heart rate was too high for PT; however, if she had been allowed to walk that day, she would have likely had her panic attack in the hallway, on a portable vent, without Ann present. It was frustrating that we missed PT, but maybe it was a blessing in disguise. I reminded her of how far she had come and that just a month earlier she might have hyperventilated and blacked out. I kissed her on the forehead and told her I was so proud of her.

The next day, as she mentally prepared for her PT session, she wanted another dose of Ativan. With three hours to reset before PT, she agreed to sleep while I inquired about the medication. I hoped she would just fall asleep before any chemical assistance arrived so we could skip it altogether. I made it happen by brushing her hair for about forty-five minutes while simultaneously finding *Avengers: Age of Ultron* show times.

Though she was able to relax enough to be ready for PT with no Ativan, we started to walk and had problems after 50 feet. A low blood sugar of 35 mg/dL shortened the session. This was not only dangerous, but it meant the end of physical therapy. This week she had completed only two walks and she was at her best for only one of them. Her one-time personal record of 300 feet seemed far away, and the target goal of 500 feet was even farther.

Pittsburgh would require a full-week evaluation and at best, she had only been able to string together a few good consecutive days. I told myself we would just have to take it as it comes since there was nothing more we could do to prepare. I hoped that much like our missed PT session the day before, things would work out for the best even if I could not envision it at the time. I worked to clear my mind of it for two hours and twenty-two minutes while the Avengers defeated

Ultron and our realm was safe yet again.

Lesson 24: Don't be discouraged if you fall short. A failure today may be a blessing in disguise.

CHAPTER 15

Keep Running

May came quickly and Norm arrived a day before the half marathon. I think he expected we would have more time to shop, get our packets, and prep for the event, but I was happy to get out for a few hours. When we finally left for dinner, he commented that it had been a long day between the hospital and the errands, but taking a few hours to do things for me was a nice break from the norm (but not from *The* Norm). This was the closest I got to a day off and I was enjoying it.

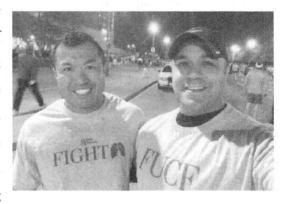

While getting our packets, I ran into a few of my colleagues from work and some brought up the situation with Rebecca while others did not. I was not sure which I preferred. I was open to talking about it but I did not want to go into too much detail and make them feel awkward. The answer to how she was doing would vary depending on what they knew. I had learned to keep my answers focused on the next steps and our hopes of getting accepted at Pittsburgh.

The race was nothing unusual and I started slow and planned to increase my speed over the course of the race. Norm decided to slow down and run with me instead of competing at his normal pace. We had no problems until he stopped for his third bathroom break because clearly, this grown man had the bladder of an adolescent girl.

When he attempted to catch up to me, he was clearly unaware of my amazing conditioning and raw speed. As my speed increased, he questioned whether or not he had missed me, so he was jogging forward and backward to find me on the course while I was winning. A post-race searching ensued and we missed each other at every turn: the finish line, the bag check, the medical tent, the car. We were like two kids lost at the fair. We eventually found each other, had a celebratory beer and I dropped him back at the airport. It had passed so quickly but my first half marathon was a nice accomplishment in the midst of everything that was happening.

Back at the hospital, Bec was having a sleepy day. She had smooth talked the doctor into increasing her dose of Ativan, resulting in her being out cold all morning. She was sleeping when I arrived but asked about the race as soon as she woke up. I knew I would be explaining it again in an hour which was okay with me because this was a story I would repeat regardless.

Since Bec had no voice, she would knock on the closest hard surface to get my attention. I normally did not mind hopping up to help with any random thing. But after lugging my 225-pound body for 13.1 miles, I was exhausted and really dreading the sound. It seemed like every time I would get settled in my chair I would hear that knock again. She would summon me to come over and I would tell her, "I can read your lips just as well from over here," all the while hoping that whatever it was would not require too much energy.

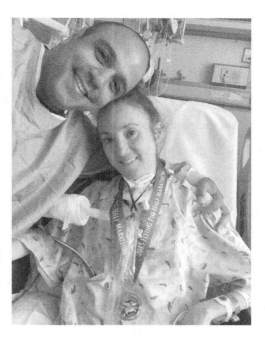

Bec had slept so much earlier in the day that she was wide awake. I had tried to leave but she looked up with little worried wrinkles on her forehead and asked me not to leave. She liked to be tucked in. After a late dinner, 10 p.m. was the earliest I could get out of there which felt particularly late since I had woken up at 4 a.m. for the race. I was tired, but looking at Becca understood that I should be thankful for what I could do. I was worn out because I was capable of running that distance on a beautiful day with a good friend. I did not have to struggle for every breath while dreading a life-threatening surgery as a best case scenario. With that reminder sitting right there in front of me, it was hard to feel sorry for myself for too long.

Lesson 25: Try not to complain. Somebody always has it worse. Particularly, try not to complain to them.

Each PT session was critical, but by this point, Rebecca had missed several PT appointments due to her tachycardia. Her heart rate would be normal in the morning then climb over the course of the day. Since PT was at 2:30 in the afternoon, we seemed to always be walking the line between acceptable and unacceptable ranges. I suggested we do physical therapy earlier so we could avoid that situation all together. Everyone agreed but by the implementation day, Becca had no recollection of this and complained that it was too early. She wanted to nap this time. She was so adamant that they suggested doing it the next day. Normally, I tried to convince her logically but with the pressure of the pending qualification I took a different route. I could see that she really did not want to and all I wanted to do was to let her rest, but you can't always get what you want.

"It has been a tough month," I told her. "You are only averaging two to three sessions per week and we've hit a plateau. There are a lot of things that are out of your control, but this is not one of them. I know you're tired, and I know it sucks but we are at a critical point. We can be headed out to Pittsburgh any day for evaluation and we need you to be as ready as you can be. If you're not healthy enough, don't walk. If you're having a panic attack then we deal with that as it comes and hope that doesn't stop us again. But if you're just tired, even extremely tired, you need to get out there and do your therapy. You can sleep any time before or after it but you get precious few appointments a week that we can participate in so we have to take full advantage of that! This is your only job right now, to rest, eat, and do therapy. You can do the other two any time of every day but there are only five opportunities a week for PT."

It was an impassioned plea but also a tough expectation. I could not understand what she was going through. But this was not me judging her, it was a reality check. Becca worked harder than anyone and I rarely had to push her, but this could not be optional. She listened, considered it seriously for a few moments, then agreed to get up and walk. There were very few moments where I was this proud of her. We called PT back in and off we went. She had a solid walk that day at 250 feet.

Her challenge was monumental. The odds were against her just to get listed. If that happened, the one-year survival rate of 80 percent was optimistic for her. Not qualifying would mean that she would never come home. The choice was clear...shitty but clear.

I awoke the following morning to Rebecca's cat purring and kneading my neck affectionately with her claws. As I dragged myself out of bed I could feel a familiar ache from my back. It would occasionally act up because of a herniated disk and the subsequent surgery I had in college. I limped around the house prepping the coffee, Bec's yogurt, and my breakfast. By the time I rushed out of the house, it was already 10:30. I arrived to see Becca sleeping soundly. Ativan had already been administered which was never a good sign. I tried to get rid of the thought that if I arrived earlier I might have kept her calm or talked her into a smaller dose.

She awoke for a few minutes and I showed her the card and the latest batch of gluten-free cookies my mom had sent. She suddenly started to cry which was not her common response to baked goods.

She told me that the cookies reminded her that her own mom did not do things like that for her. The fact that she had not sent Rebecca a card did not go unnoticed. "I feel like she doesn't even care," she told me. The only thing Brenda had really done was text Rebecca with some frequency but even that stopped for a couple of weeks after our prickly discussion about the fundraiser. I found myself defending Brenda again as I explained that everybody handles things differently but she could be sure that Brenda loved her.

As Bec dozed, I got to work. There was much to do that day, including phone calls and preparations for the transfer. I was about to add a few more calls to the list. Pat, the social worker at the Drake Center, stopped in to discuss some issues with my insurance. Aetna was looking to transfer Rebecca out of the Drake Center to another type of long-term care facility. This new facility would have less of a focus on preparing Rebecca for transplant and more of a focus on maintaining her care. She did not say those words specifically, but I was pretty sure we were talking about hospice care. This risk had been looming in the background since the initial tour of the Drake Center when the nurse told us that insurance often put time limits on how long patients were permitted to stay there. This was a step in the wrong direction, focused on comfort and maintenance rather than on improvement and preparation for transplant.

As I worked through my call list, I moved through it one item at a time. A couple of hours into it there was a knock on her door. I looked up and it was Pat again. She had been working on her end and things were progressing, in a good way. We were potentially a day or two away from transferring to UPMC.

As she spoke to me about my travel coverage, the pulmonologists walked up. We were ready to go and just needed a bed to open up in the Pittsburgh MICU and to lock down the logistics. The pulmonologists that were rounding at the time were actually the same ones that had rounds in the MICU when Rebecca was admitted on New Year's Eve.

UPMC had been told that Rebecca had walked 250 feet the day before. It turned out that this was good and that there was not a minimum distance requirement at UPMC, they looked at the full picture. I was thrilled she had pushed herself that day! Everything seemed to be falling in line.

I went back to Becca's room and paced back and forth hoping she would wake up and I could tell her. I did not know what to do with myself. I had to go home and pack because I would be riding in the transport with her very soon. I also knew I would want to stay there until her PT session so I could give her a pep talk beforehand. I would also need to buy cat food and arrange for pet care while I was gone. I should give at least one neighbor the keys to our house in case of emergency. I had a day or two to do all of this. It was GO time.

With all of the excitement of the transfer, I really wanted to siphon that energy into a great walk. I was hoping that when she did wake up, she would be more relaxed and mentally ready for PT. I thought maybe a great pep talk like the day before would be just what was needed. After she woke up, I told her the good news about Pittsburgh. She was groggy but managed to make the keen observation that "they weren't joking." Indeed they were not.

I was getting myself pretty excited. I told her how great it was that she walked 250 feet the day before and that the doctors had communicated this to UPMC. The fact that we would only be here a few more days meant that we would have to take advantage of every walk and really push it. She stopped me right there and told me that she was not going to push it. She would do what she could and I was making her nervous. Well crap, my pep talk was only working on me.

As I went about my tasks of transferring her from the bed to the commode to her chair, prepping her food, asking for cold milk, and rearranging the furniture, my back was killing me. The pain must have affected my demeanor because after finally getting her situated in the recliner, she asked if I was mad at her. While I tried convincing her I was not mad, I was thinking about PT because Ann was not there. Meanwhile, her stomach began bothering her from lunch and she looked miserable. So now she was physically in pain and dreading her PT session (probably even more so because of me). To top it off, Ann would not be there to operate the vent.

When the time came for therapy, she had her game face on. I could tell she was fighting through tiredness and anxiety. We got out into the hallway and she pushed forward. She only got 156 feet but she worked incredibly hard to get there. She could not physically go any further and we could see that she was let down by what she did. It became even clearer to me at that point how hard these walks had been for her. We got back to the room and I told her that I was proud of her. This was the first time she had been able to walk with an RT other than Ann. This was the first time she had ever walked three days in a row. This was the longest total weekly distance she had managed in over a month and it was only Wednesday. The praise seemed to make her feel a little better and I was happy to avoid an "I'm not proud of myself" moment.

Knowing that it was snoozer time, I started packing up the room with plans to start bringing some things home and pack up for the next adventure. It's amazing how much stuff we had accumulated. I would stop at home to get a bag going there and then come back to tuck her in. I did not know how long I was packing for, so I made up for it by packing an excessive amount of underwear. I was cautious not to pull a Becca Pack Job which entails planning at least three options for every possible scenario. She had done this on our Maui trip and if memory serves me, there was an entire bag dedicated to flip flops. In addition to including generous underwear supplies, my packing philosophy centered on gym gear, jeans, and an assumption that any other issues would work themselves out.

I came in and saw the prep cart for her trach change. The first thing she said was that she wanted versed this time and that they needed to give her enough. She held up three fingers to represent her demands. The pulmonologist came in and Bec was already fired up, annoyed that they were talking in the hallway and excluding her. She told him that she needed versed and would refuse the procedure if she did not get it. She was learning the system. She told them that she needed 3 mg—smaller amounts do not work on her. He gave her two but had some more prepped in case she needed it. After a minute or so, he asked how it was working. Rebecca sat there with a look that perfectly combined defiance and sarcasm (one that I'd become quite familiar with over the years). She threw both hands up, "Does it look like it's working? I'm wide awake!" Welcome to my world, doctor...

In order to stay out of the way, I stood at the bottom of her bed and held her toes. I would periodically try to say something encouraging letting her know I was there. Unfortunately, I had a front row seat to the whole procedure, blood and all. She started coughing right from the start. I could see them pull the old trach out and all of the secretions were around it. As they inserted the new trach, I could see her say, "Ouch, ouch, ouch," as she tightened her fists and winced. A little blood started to dribble down, not a large amount, but enough. There are three times when a front row seat sucks: a class you're not prepared for, a mean comedian, and a trach change.

In the meantime, the transfer was moving forward. I got a call from Pat and she told me that the transport company would want some money in advance. I asked how much and the answer was "all of it." Due to the distance we had to go, it was in the ballpark of $9,000. That was a nice little surprise in the ninth hour. The transport company was not willing to work with the insurance company in the same way everyone else did. They had me over a barrel. I spoke with Aetna to confirm my coverage, that they would reimburse me, and to see if they had recommendations. They gave me a list of questions to ask the transport company but by the time I got over to see Pat, she had things under control and said she would let me know if she needed me to do anything. Now it was time to wait.

Aetna approved us for three days in Pittsburgh. I had been under the impression that we would go there, get evaluated, and then find out if we were staying. It did not make sense to send Rebecca back before they knew if she would be listed. She would have to suffer through two additional five-hour drives that could be avoided all together if she stayed there. That would result in an additional $18,000 of transport costs that Aetna would have to cover at 80 percent. They would not save any money by bringing her back sooner because they would have to pay for her care wherever she was. I laid this out in an email and hoped that common sense would prevail. Maybe we could convince the doctor that Bec couldn't travel again because of her anxiety...but I was getting ahead of myself.

Friday was focused on locking down all of the details for her trip to Pittsburgh. The first transport company had fallen through so I sat down with Pat and we called Aetna again along with several transport companies. I was surprised at how hard it was to find a service that would be willing to transport a person on a vent. One lady told me right off the bat that we would have to pay in advance. She had a bit of an attitude and acted like that would scare me off. As she rushed to get off the phone with me, I told her that was what I had expected and asked how much it would cost. She fumbled around a bit then told me they would not be able to do it. I figured I would get in a little parting shot. I asked her if she knew of any companies that might have the capability; she did not. So I said, "I suppose I'll need to find a larger national company with much more capability but thank you anyway." Ultimately, we did lock down a service for Monday morning,

7 a.m. Things were moving in the right direction and I was thrilled!

It was particularly difficult leaving that night because she was tired and uncomfortable. It was about 8:30 and she asked me to stay until her RT came in. I called and found out that he was saving her for last because he wanted to spend more time with her since her lungs had been more "junky" that day. He would probably be in around 10 p.m. which sounded good to me but less so to Rebecca. I felt a little guilty playing my trump card of wanting to eat dinner but I kind of...wanted to eat dinner.

It was still a tough balance of being there for Bec but also having a little time for me. I could reason with myself that it was okay but the guilt would never truly go away. I needed time to myself to keep my sanity but I would think back to January when I prayed for just one more conversation with her. I had prayed for just a little more time and those prayers were answered. Yet I was still leaving when she wanted me there. It felt almost ungrateful. I always felt I was sleeping too late and leaving too early. I would go to the gym and hope that she slept while I was gone so she did not sit there by herself, alone and bored. I would get to the room and hope she was just waking up though it was typically the opposite. I continued to push her Kindle on her because I wanted to feel that she was occupied with something when I was not there. She would often forget where I had gone which made me feel worse. Then, within fifteen minutes of arriving she would be sound asleep and I would sit in the chair and play Sudoku while sneaking glances at her.

As I tucked Rebecca in that night I was looking forward to

going to the new burger joint near our house and rewarding myself with some nice craft beer. I headed straight there and found a good spot at the bar. I chatted with a couple next to me about college basketball. I told them neat facts about UConn, they told me neat facts about Kentucky, and we both expressed our dislike for Duke. It was a nice break. I went home and decided to continue my sampling of craft beer and even included some Miller Lite, for comparison sake. My conclusion was that each and every one of them contained alcohol and that alcohol made you sleep late.

It was almost noon when I got to her room. The RT told me that her CO_2 was high and I could tell by her tone that it was concerning. It had been 118 mEq/L when they first checked but had dropped to 109 by the time I had arrived. Her numbers had not been over 100 since they had given her the paralytic in January. The X-ray did not show anything so they tried to clear out some mucus using a process called cough assist. It used added positive pressure then switched to negative pressure to dislodge potential mucus plugs. They also used a process called lavage where they put saline in her lungs then suctioned it out in hopes it would thin out the secretions. Her O_2 had been turned up from 40 percent to 50 percent and her tidal volumes (volume of air that is inhaled and exhaled in a single breath) were increased as well. I wondered if this would affect our Pittsburgh travel.

Hopefully it was just due to the volume settings being too low and not because her lungs were getting worse. It felt like they were. Her respiratory rate had been higher for a month and her O_2 sats were creeping down, particularly in the past week. From what I could tell, her secretions had been getting thicker. As I sat there watching her numbers, I could see her pressure was now at 50 cmH_2O versus the 15 cmH_2O from a couple of weeks ago.

I woke her up for suctioning and she was not too pleased with me. She told me—quite annoyed—that she was sleeping well. I went down twice with the tube and by the third she informed me that this was the last one. With all of the secretions I was able to suction, I was expecting her pressure to go down but it did not. I needed to stop looking at it because watching her numbers was the opposite of therapeutic.

I still had not sent an update to everyone on the current situation since I felt that it would only stress everyone at this point. If it passed, I could send a note explaining what happened and how it was resolved. It would be just another victory for Bec. If it got worse I would tell everyone as well. But I really hated to send those texts. I knew it felt horrible to hear bad news and be far away in no position to do anything about it. I suppose I could not do much about it either but it did no good to stress them out further. I would just wait and hope that nobody asked me how Bec was doing today. I gave as much thought to the updates that I sent as I did to the updates I did not.

Lesson 26: Those who are not there do not need to know every detail in real time. Instead, just be present.

After the next blood draw, Becca's CO_2 level was still over 100 mEq/L. This was becoming more serious so the doctor spoke to the head of pulmonology at the hospital. They decided to send us back to the MICU. They thought it was a mucus plug because she had no fever and her white count was not elevated over her baseline. The pulmonologists at the MICU might have the capability to remove a plug if that was the cause.

I feared another bronchoscopy. After the last one she had become very sensitive to position changes which would cause her to sats to drop suddenly and drastically. It was right before she hit her lowest point and was placed on the paralytic in January. Maybe it was not caused by the bronch but it got me nervous nonetheless. I reminded myself that she was much more sick back then. There was no reason to think this could not be resolved and even though we were moving at the speed of "hospital," there were intelligent people managing her care that not only understood her situation, but genuinely cared for her.

CHAPTER 16

ICU but I Can't Quit You

The earliest the transport could arrive was 7:30 p.m. and it was going to be a late night. We arrived in the MICU and had one of the same nurses from January. So many people told Rebecca how much better she looked. She, of course, did not recognize anyone. It was like being a kid and having a parent's friend tell you how big you got and then show you how tall you were when they last saw you.

The night started with more X-rays, blood gases, and airway clearance. The pulmonologists came by a couple of times to talk about diagnostic options but admitted that they were not sure why her CO_2 was so high. It was creeping down but way too slowly. We decided on doing a bronch. Rebecca asked for sedation and was demanding 4 mg of versed. That was the number in her head and the doctors could not talk her out of it. I was on the fence of whether or not I should try convincing her doctors because I knew that it would knock her out for hours. I hated to see her panic but that stuff was liquid amnesia.

By this point, it was midnight and all they could get me was a crappy uncomfortable chair. My car was across town, my back still hurt, and I was still a little hungover from my craft beer celebration the night before. My green Shit Happens colon cleanse bag was on the floor next to me and was starting to look pretty rough. It had coffee stains on it, a hole, and some of the stitching was unravelling. I felt like I needed to dress well when I was carrying it or I ran the risk of looking like a homeless person. My toothbrush was packed in the luggage in the car and I really just wanted a snoozer.

My mind kept wandering back to the bronch. I had informed family about this whole ordeal but no one else. I wanted to get the message out there so I could show Rebecca the flood of support, but at this point I was cautious about posting anything negative online. The fear was that UPMC would see it and it would somehow damage our chance at acceptance. I also worried that even if she knocked this issue down, it could wear her out and impact her evaluation in the coming week.

It was good that she got the sedation because this bronch was much more intrusive than the last few had been. They took a biopsy which I expected but it was still a surprise to see the blood being suctioned from her lungs. They put a tongue protector in her mouth and brought the scope through there as well. They checked the trachea in the area of contact with the trach balloon. All of these evaluations showed no major problems. This was both good and bad because we did not want to find a major issue but we wanted to find out what was going on.

It was about 1:30 a.m. when they finished the procedure. During rounds the next morning, they talked through the potential causes and settled on a new infection. Her PCO_2 (carbon dioxide partial pressure) had dropped to 96 mmHg, so it was still high but kept slowly creeping downward. Her blood pressure was 64/40 mmHg (far below the target of 120/80 mmHg). Fluids helped bring it back up but in the meantime she was quite disoriented. At one point she pointed across the room laughing at something. It was nice that someone was having a good time. She had so much to say but she was not moving her lips very much so she was hard to understand. She took about ten minutes to tell me that she used up all of her vacation time. I told her, "Yes, dear, we've got to get you back to work soon."

I could hear trach noises all day which sounded like a cross between a moan and a honk. For a temporary fix, we could move the vent tubes and adjust the amount of air in the cuff but this only lasted a few seconds. The leaking air would sometimes come while she was saying something then instantly she would have this robotic sounding voice. She was napping most of the day but she would wake herself up from all of the talking she was doing in her sleep. Her CO_2 levels and pH were both continuing to head in the right direction. I left to run some errands and when I got back I heard a couple of her doctors talking about a lady demanding versed. I was not sure what was going on but I was guessing that lady was Rebecca.

I got to the room and she told me they were planning another trach change. They believed air was leaking out of the trach balloon. They explained how the balloon had stretched out her trach and how her cuff pressures were already super high. I had heard all of this before and really did not want to hear it again but all I could do was hope it was a problem with the device itself. It was critical that we get her "right" before the morning because we wanted the doctors to have no reason to delay her travel to UPMC.

They completed the procedure and not thirty seconds later, we heard the familiar sound of air leaking. All of that fuss and it resolved nothing. As the doctors started to look at other trachs and speak about consulting with the ENTs, it looked like this could become our next major impediment. At this point, Bec was out cold from the versed and I was of the mindset that I did not care if there was a leak. She was oxygenating, getting her volumes, and her blood gases were continuing to improve. As far as I was concerned, they could deal with this at UPMC.

As the RT placed the dressing around her trach, the sound suddenly stopped. By pulling it out an inch or so to work, the cuff moved to a different spot and the leak went away. I'm not sure why none of us thought of this before the procedure but no matter — problem solved. Let's give her a blanket, turn off the lights, and not touch her until tomorrow!

I was so excited to move to the next step that morning. I packed my bag with clothes for both of us, the laptop bag had all of our paperwork, and the cooler had a ton of food. We were only approved for three days but I knew that logic, along with my smooth talking, would prevail and insurance would approve an extension through the listing decision.

I took an Uber to the hospital and left my car at home. I had too much nervous energy to sit still, so I split my time between bouncing alternating knees and pacing. As the time ticked away, I waited for the doctors to give the final green light because the transport was already on its way! When Gina, the social worker, stopped in, I quickly learned that she was unaware of our transport to Pittsburgh. I instantly worried that the weekend staff did not follow up properly and the ambulance was erroneously heading to the Drake Center. Reality was worse.

It turned out that after Rebecca was transferred to the MICU, she was diagnosed with pneumonia and the Pittsburgh evaluation was cancelled with plans to re-initiate discussions when and if she recovered. The transport was not coming. It was incredibly frustrating to say the least. There was such a narrow window where Becca's condition was concerned and any opportunity missed could potentially be a big deal. To top it off, her friend Stephanie was flying out from Maine to surprise her at UPMC and now she would be sitting in a strange city by herself while Rebecca was here. I could see everything we had worked for start to crumble.

Her new attending, Dr. Renee Hebbeler-Clark, disagreed with the diagnosis but it was already in the file so our only chance was to reverse the diagnosis. She noted that Becca had no elevated white count, no fever, and X-rays showed her lungs looked a thousand times better than during her previous pneumonia. Fortunately, her pulmonologist from the night before agreed. Our chance at a Pittsburgh evaluation was riding on this one diagnosis. Her symptoms also cleared up after the bronch and some additional airway clearance. She was adamant that Rebecca did not have pneumonia and thankfully got the official diagnosis reversed. It was a huge relief, but we still had a ways to go. All we could do was wait and hope that she stayed healthy for another day. She was still very tired which I suspected was because of the versed she had received the night before and the overall energy she expended fighting this latest battle in her lungs.

In fact, as I sat there trying to see the silver lining, it became clear that she would not have had a great showing that day if she had made the trip. Perhaps this was another blessing in disguise. We knew that Pittsburgh was her last real chance at a transplant and that this evaluation would determine her survival. As long as it was just one more day, maybe more rest would do her some good.

I hated sending the text update to everyone since we were all so excited for some forward progress. I sent out the note and my phone was blowing up with messages from everyone, mostly asking about how she was doing and the new plan. Brenda asked me for her new address. I flashed back to the last address request where her presumed intent was a surprise move to Cincinnati. I could not stop her from moving but I was not about to do her more favors if she was planning to blindside us again. I just KNEW she had the same plan. The best card I could play was to demonstrate that a visit this early was a bad investment, so I told everyone about the three-day insurance window and did not expand on my ongoing efforts to get it extended. The speed of her response supported my theory.

May 11, 2015 Text from Brenda: *Returning Wednesday??? Back to Cincinnati? Then back to Pittsburg again??*

I told her that it came down to insurance requirements. Maybe she was simply confused by the logistics, but her fast emotional response convinced me that she was secretly planning something. Had she told me she would like to visit, I would have provided a more detailed explanation. But if it was a secret, then she was on her own. I had come to realize that our hospital room was even more than a second home for us, it was essentially our bedroom. To show up unannounced showed a lack of respect and was an intrusion. I was not sure what was in store, but I worried so much about the pending week that I preferred to avoid Brenda's drama.

Soon it was too late to get a transport for that day and possibly even the next day. Even if we could, UPMC suggested she transfer as early as possible in the morning because of the three day evaluation time limit. I had previously planned to address the duration of stay when we arrived at UPMC but it would be easier to arrange a transport if the time of day did not matter. I called Aetna and began working on them, leveraging that they would need to pay for her care wherever she was and that they could save the cost of some back and forth travel if approved. I got an encouraging response over the phone but it would be another day before they could give official approval.

There were a few people milling around in the area outside of her room. I assumed they were there for another patient until they started gowning up. A lady from physical therapy started talking to Rebecca asking if she was ready to get up and walk. It was driven by a request from UPMC and felt very rushed. We had no chance to give Becca any anti-anxiety medication. Luckily she had become much better at managing her anxiety. In fact this time, I was much more anxious than she was, but there was no choice.

They were not using the portable vent settings that we used at the Drake Center. The RT told me that they did not have those settings. I had them. She needed the best shot to succeed and if I needed to be a pain in the ass, I would be. Except...as I made her walk me through the settings, I realized that there was not actually a big difference. The only difference was the respiratory rate at 26 versus 24 bpm. When I saw that, I just shut up and let them do their thing.

Bec on the other hand, handled it like a pro. She switched to the portable vent with no visible anxiety. She sat up on the side of the bed and caught her breath then she up and walked 152 feet with no issues. She knew what she needed to do and she was on a mission!

They returned her vent to previous settings but she struggled to stay there. As the day went on, her sats continued to run right on the bottom of the range, dipping into the high 80s every few minutes. I left that night completely worn out. She was borderline but her condition often changed so quickly that she could rebound completely the next day, or she could be worse. I got home and all I could think about was the strength she would need to get through the next day...and the next few days. This was her chance and she was not at her best.

It was overwhelming. As soon as I walked through the door I started to pray. I remember dropping down to my knees in my family room and praying that God would give her strength of body, mind, and spirit. I prayed that He would lay His healing hands on her and give her the energy to do her best and that she get accepted. I had no energy for dinner so I just went upstairs and tried to get to sleep. This was momentous for me because I had never before been too tired to eat.

CHAPTER 17

Planes, Trains, and Automobiles...
Except for Trains

I arrived at the hospital all ramped up because this was the day and 7 a.m. was the time! At about ten after, I called Ohio Ambulance to see where they were and I was told they were twenty minutes out due to traffic. Several calls and an hour later they arrived. One of them strutted in with the look and rebellious eyes of Joan Jett; she had an attitude right from the start. When our RT, Bridgette, asked her to put on a mask Joan gave some story about being claustrophobic. I was hoping that she was the driver and would not be back there with Becca because I knew she would take it off and we were going to clash. Bec looked at me as if to say, "I don't know about these two..."

As they tried to hook her up, Bridgette helped and I got a few looks from her that told me she was also less than impressed with Joan. When they started having problems with an O_2 alarm, Joan insisted their vent was fine. After calling in some help to troubleshoot, the vent was just not working and it occurred to me that this transport might not happen.

Joan was loud to begin with and was getting frustrated which did not help the situation. When Dr. Hebbeler-Clark came in, I could tell she had been talking to Bridgette and she put a stop to the transfer then and there. Right in front of them, she told us that Becca needed to travel by air transport with a crew that was more qualified and capable. I was relieved. The transport team slinked off (presumably to listen to rock and roll from a jukebox, baby) and did not say a word to us. Good riddance!

With the B-team gone, we had to secure a new way to get to Pittsburgh. The previous day, Gina called sixteen different places to book this company and now we were back at square one. I felt bad for Rebecca's friend, Stephanie, who had traveled out to Pittsburgh to meet us. She had to decide if it made sense to come down to Cincinnati and that was all based on my recommendation. Gina had told me about one option but the company did not take insurance and we would have to cover about $18,000. Not great but we wouldn't rule it out completely.

As she got back on the phone, all I could do was watch from my room and wait. I didn't know what to do with myself. I texted Stephanie that maybe it would be better if she drove down but that I would confirm it once I spoke with Gina again. I would hate for her to come all that way and not be able to see Rebecca. I went on Facebook posting a snapshot of a comically large (yet somehow not so funny) $613,000+ bill I had received from the hospital. At this point, the whole situation just felt ridiculous.

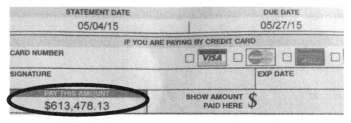

I heard what sounded like Gina saying something in an excited tone. I could not make it out but I saw her on the phone outside of the room and waited to see if it had to do with us. About ten minutes later, I saw her walking to the room with a phone and a spring in her step. She had found a transport!

I spoke to them on the phone and they sounded like they had their shit together. It was a company that would take us by ambulance to a small local airport, transport us to Pittsburgh on a jet, and then bring us to the bed at UPMC. I fought the urge to hug Gina because I was still wearing my isolation gown...but I was thrilled! Now, instead of pacing from anxiety, I was pacing from excitement!

It would be great to get Bec to Pittsburgh but we would need a good showing when we got there. She was sleepy and I had no black market connections for speed or any other uppers. I guess we would just stick with Plan A and hope that sleeping off those sedatives and recovering from her procedures would be enough. A fine plan but one with no pizzazz...

The air transport team arrived and it was night and day from Ms. Jett's team that morning. They were extremely professional and had an air of competency about them. They also had a sense of urgency and we raced through the Cincinnati downtown with ambulance sirens singing.

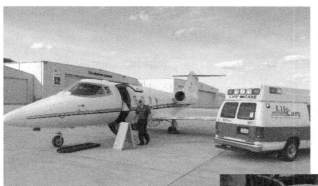

We got to the jet and they loaded her up with no issues. I could see how nervous she was but she was able to concentrate on keeping herself calm. Had this been a month before, it would have surely meant a panic attack but Becca had improved on so many fronts. She kept asking for Ativan and they listened to her, reasoned with her, and administered multiple doses while being careful not to give her too much. This reinforced the notion that the hurdles of the morning happened for a reason. I knew this was a thousand times better than taking a road trip with the band. I brought a flower for her to hold onto in the jet and sat with my hand on her foot for the short flight.

As we entered the hospital in Pittsburgh, Stephanie was there to meet us and we all squeezed onto the elevator. I got a half-smile from Bec, and then I pointed at her friend and said, "You've got a visitor!" I saw her process it for a second then a huge smile came across her face. She was so excited! What a great pick-me-up for Bec at such a critical point. Bec reached for her hand, and then pulled it toward her mouth to kiss it. The vent tube got in the way but that wasn't going to stop her. I knew this would help her morale for days!

The next day, we anxiously awaited the first transplant team doctor. When Dr. Bruce Johnson arrived, Bec had just transferred to the chair and was sitting up, looking alert. This was timed perfectly. He asked why she had not been approved at the other hospitals. Our concerns were eased one issue at a time. The vent did not concern him if she had good muscle mass and could walk a reasonable distance. After training for 500 feet (for Michigan) it looked like all she would need to do was 100 feet. The *B. cepacia* was not a roadblock because she had not cultured it since 2010. He commented that most of the bad bacteria would come out with the old lungs.

He asked about her liver and kidney issues and she told him how they were under control. He explained the transplant risks, medications, follow ups, and life expectancies. Rebecca was alert and sharp the whole time. Bec was shining that morning. I could not have hoped that this would happen any other time or in any other way. He told us that Rebecca looked like a very good candidate. It was Wednesday and they would not have their formal review until the following Tuesday. The surgeons and other transplant team members would have a chat with her, but this was a fantastic start!

Bec was complaining quite a bit about pain that day, mostly headaches but stomach pain as well. When her trach started making noise again, I could see her frustration rising. She demanded to know why it was doing that. I tried to calm her a bit and reminded her how it made more noise when she breathed heavily. It was not long before she started to get upset. It was so overwhelming and the pain only compounded the issue. As she started to tear up, I sat down next to her and told her I had a good feeling about this place and that everything that happened today was positive. I gave her as much of a hug as I could around the trach tubes. I put my cheek on the side of her face, pulled her close, and told her how proud I was of her and how she did a great job today. As she calmed down, she asked me to brush her hair. It did the trick as she closed her eyes and nodded with approval. It had already been a long road but we still had some tough hurdles ahead of us.

The culture in this hospital was a bit different from Cincinnati. They asked me to leave as soon as we arrived to "clean her up." Begrudgingly, I left and waited for the call that I could return. The next night, they decided to change her room and I was kicked out while they prepared to bag her and told me again to wait for the call. I tried to warn them about her anxiety but they did not really understand. By this point I had fully become an overprotective mom and I was embracing it. When the transfer was complete, they forgot to call me and I missed a text from Rebecca asking me to come back. Fortunately, we had a code, if I did not respond quickly enough to a text, I told her to call. It would be enough to bring my attention to the text and I would respond ASAP (Deere).

Her call alerted me to a text that she had arrived and was looking for me. Since they had forgotten, she was in her new room scared and alone. When I arrived she had a cool towel on her head, her face was red, and her eyes were glassy. She looked very concerned and asked where I had been. As I spoke to her and tried to calm her, I knew this would be a rough night. She did not like the fact that she had all male caregivers and because of the partially closed door she told me that they were trying to close her in. I knew it was just the anxiety talking but I dreaded the next day and how she would hold up when I was not with her.

She was so apologetic when she asked me not to leave that night. I told her it was no big deal but I was not allowed to sleep in the new room with her like at UC. I would stay with her until she fell asleep then I would be right around the corner in the waiting room...just a text away. She agreed to it and apologized again for asking. She said she could not do this without me. I told her she would never have to. It was not the first time she had said that and it made me feel both good and bad simultaneously. It felt great to be there for her when she needed me but it felt horrible that she needed me in this way. Neither of us ever had the "Why me?" type of mentality but it was so tough to see her in this position.

It was all so surreal. We were in a strange place, had all new health challenges, and had no idea of what to expect next. I could trust that we had made the best decisions in getting to that point so there could be no regrets. If I was going to get through this situation with no regrets I had to be the man she needed me to be. That meant staying in the hospital when I knew she needed me to and it meant giving her the confidence that I was an unshakable fixture in her life that she could count on. I did not have to comply with all of her wishes, just the ones that gave her that type of support.

It seemed like Bec was a little disoriented but I attributed it to the anxiety. As I sat in the room waiting for her to fall asleep, the nurse requested a urine sample. When Bec got on the bed pan and was trying to pee, it lasted for over fifteen minutes. I kept asking if she had gone. The answer was always, "No,"...until it was, "There's no toilet paper." She had been unsuccessful for so long I had thought she was just being proactive. It turns out she had gone. This was a little odd but not alarming yet. She went right to sleep afterward and I was almost ready for my "comfy" recliner in the waiting room.

About fifteen minutes later, I went to give a last look before slipping out and her eyes were open. She was asking me how she was going to package all twenty-four candles on the shelves behind her. When I told her there were no candles she looked at me like I was intentionally trying to piss her off and that she had no patience for it. With my iPad camera reversed, I showed her the room behind her and how there were not twenty-four candles requiring packaging and shipment. She told me she must have dreamt that she was back at UConn and had twelve candles to package. Ambien. It must be due to friggin' Ambien.

I finally made it back to the waiting room and started to relax. After about forty-five minutes of web surfing and Sudoku, I was getting sleepy. Just then, the phone rang. It was her nurse asking me to return. I expected to see her anxious when I got back but instead, she was on a mission. "Help me get dressed," she told me "I'm ready to go." I asked where and she said she wanted to sit up on the side of the bed. "When will the ambulance be here?"

"There's no ambulance coming, dear. You are exactly where you're supposed to be. We're in Pittsburgh and you handled the traveling great. I'm so proud of you."

She started to nod and I knew she accepted what I said at some level because she started to relax. I told her that she was the bravest person I knew. She looked at me like I was a snake oil salesman, so I explained it. "Being brave does not mean you aren't scared. Being brave means you do what you have to in spite of that fear. Look how you handled the transport here. I saw you focused and working hard to stay calm and in control. You handled multiple crews and a lot of activity. You handled two ambulance rides and a flight. You handled being admitted in a new hospital while dealing with a lot of pain from your worsening headaches. You are amazing and I'm proud of you."

Like an English teacher, she seemed to accept that because I supported my statement. I asked her if she wanted to read and she shook her head no. "Well I guess you can go to sleep if you really want," and she nodded *yes*. She was getting loopy again and this time she did not have high CO_2 or a recent versed dose. I started to think back to ICU delirium. I sat there thinking that it was a hell of a time for her to lose her mind. I needed to have some theory so I could calm my mind and go to sleep. Do I try to get her some help or do I just keep my mouth shut until we're listed?

CHAPTER 18

ICU Delirium—and I Wish You'd Stop

The morning was no different. She was incredibly tired and had trouble drinking and eating due to what appeared to be her coordination. She would hold the water bottle to her lips but come short of tipping it up enough to get the water. She would try to eat but she kept putting her fork under the edge of her plate. I really started getting concerned at this point. I checked her blood sugar again, even though I knew it would be high and not explain this behavior. There was no major change to her drug regimen that seemed like it might explain this. As the panic welled inside me, the next logical question was what to do. If I brought their attention to it, would it hurt her chances for the transplant? If I didn't, would they notice it? Which option would be worse for our chances?

She had received another blood transfusion the day before. This was the only thing that was different enough to explain it. She had not been like this after the four other ones she had received, but she was always incredibly tired the following day. This must be her new tired.

When the CF doctor arrived, I felt it would be best to bring it up but downplay it a bit and suggest my blood transfusion theory. I figured that he could chime in if he had a better one and if not, I would lay the groundwork for an acceptable, temporary reason why she was acting like this.

I brought this up to the nurse and RT as well and asked if she could get some Benadryl. That was a mixed blessing because it would make the team aware of this but it could also make her sleepier which could exacerbate the problem. As I settled on that theory, I started kicking myself for not declining the transfusion in the first place. We could have just done it a day later and she could have been at her best for the evaluation. I started to calm down a bit now that I had a theory and a plan to spread it like a ninth-grade girl gossiping about…whatever it is they gossip about. Sluts, maybe…?

The first of the transplant surgeons stopped in as Bec was waking up. He casually asked where she was coming from and she thought a bit and said "Michigan"….awww crap. He looked confused and I had a second to act.

I said to her (and him), "Yes, Michigan turned us down." Then casually threw out that we were from Cincinnati hoping he was not checking her mental state. He seemed to be okay with me answering so I just took over. He asked if she was always this sleepy and I explained how she would normally get that way after a transfusion. I just wanted her to perk up…and not say we came from Michigan! Maybe I needed to sprinkle a little crack into her water…

Adding to the bad timing for health issues, her CO_2 started to rise again (climbing to 89 mEq/L) which can also make you sleepy, a little edema was coming back, she started desatting with turns, and she had a low grade temperature. What a terrible time to have all of this happen. Not only were we there for the transplant evaluation, but Becca was a new patient so they did not have the history to see that this was a bad day. I believed that most of this was due to the transfusion. It looked like a test was planned for that day that did not require walking, which was the silver lining. I prayed that this would be short lived. I had to believe that it would work out.

The next morning was much better. Rebecca was less sleepy and less disoriented as well. Her sats had improved but her edema continued to get worse, particularly in her arms. We did a few arm exercises to help with this and to just get her moving again. Most of the evaluation was complete, but she had not walked yet. There was a PT appointment at 1 p.m. but we did not know if that was for general exercise or an evaluation. When occupational therapy (OT) came in to move her to the chair I was happy. This mirrored her routine at the Drake Center and routine was good for her anxiety.

The challenge came when they started to get her into the chair. They needed to reverse the position of the trach which basically meant disconnecting it, repositioning and reconnecting it, which I had done plenty of times before. Unfortunately, when the OT asked Bec if she wanted me to do it, Bec said she wanted the nurse. She either did not fully understand what they meant or did not remember me doing it.

As they determined the order of events for transferring her in this tight area, the plan sounded logical. As the nurse disconnected the tube, his backside pushed on the vent causing the other end to disconnect as well. He reattached the neck connection, then as he turned to address the vent it popped off her neck. All kinds of vent alarms were ringing and I could sense her stress level rising. It took what seemed like a few minutes to get it all reconnected and back in the right orientation. They stood her up and as she walked toward the chair, she tripped over one of the front casters. They were right there to catch her but her face was starting to get red. Then the tube popped off her trach again as she was asking to sit back in the bed. She was nearing another panic attack!

By the time they got her to the chair, I could see her forehead compressed with wrinkles. They were doing their best but had not experienced Bec's anxiety nor did they understand how commotion brings it on. I was so glad when they were done but Murphy's Law was in full effect. I winced when she asked for her Ativan for the first time in a few days. I knew it would knock her out just in time for PT. Even if this was not a qualifying walk, the transplant team could still inquire about the session and weigh it in their decision. However, when PT arrived, Rebecca had her game face on. She knew what she had to do because she had done it a thousand times before. Knowing that the new target was 100 feet (not 500 feet) filled both of us with confidence. She walked 220 feet with only one break and everyone seemed pleased. I was filled with pride and so happy for Bec knowing that all of that hard work had paid off. When I posted a picture of it on her site, Rachel had commented that she was walking herself right into the transplant line. That captured exactly how I felt.

It was time to leave and I was feeling accomplished. Most of the testing was done and the rest was out of our hands. Rebecca looked a bit unsettled and told me that she needed to get back to her room. This would have made way more sense if we were not already in her room. She ignored me when I told her and ordered "Get my socks!" as she propped herself up on one elbow. She was not about to sleep in the wrong bed so all she needed was her socks and she would be off to her room. Trying to get her to recognize her location, I asked if

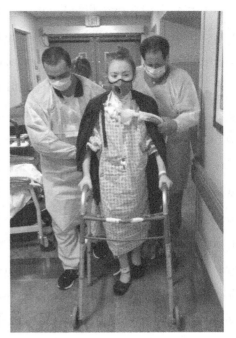

she remembered the walk earlier and reminded her that we had left from this room. As I recapped a few other events of the day, she recalled them and began to calm down. She had some incidents overnight where she was disoriented and the next night she again alerted us that she was in the wrong bed. I could no longer blame this on the transfusion...her delirium was back.

Part of the delirium treatment was to keep her more awake during the day so she could sleep at night. It was so hard for her to stay awake during the day because she was on Ativan and Seroquel for anxiety, and fentanyl and oxycodone for pain. Everything made her tired. To top it off, her body had to work extremely hard to survive. She had a breathing machine but her body still had to transfer the O_2 into her blood and the CO_2 out, it had to circulate her blood with a heart that had once failed, and it performed every movement with atrophied muscles. Whether I liked it or not, there were some legitimate reasons for all of the snoozers.

On Sunday I made the bold move of attempting to go to the gym. Though technically successful, it became clear that we needed to refine our communication a bit more. We still had our system where if she ever needed something urgently, she should text me then follow up with a call to ensure I would see it. Luckily, there was an LA Fitness nearby so I jogged a half mile to the hotel, one and a half miles to the gym, warmed up on the flat bench, and then Rebecca rang. Hoping it was nothing urgent I just spoke into the phone, probably a little too loud, narrating my actions to her and the rest of the gym knowing I was not going to get a response. Checking my texts, I see nothing and I tell her that.

May 17, 2015 Text to Bec at 1 p.m.: *Do u need something? Why did u call?*

Four minutes later she responds…

Ha

That was it.

???

Do u need me to come back?

Three minutes later I get…

Hamburgers from new place with when aldo

And she adds a bunch of concerned little emojis with a tear and blue forehead.

Did that mean temperature? She had been hot. She had never asked for hamburgers before.

If ur hot, hit ur call light and get a bag of ice and a new cool towel.

So I waited. A few minutes later, my workout was done. I could not concentrate and if this is how she was texting, she might not be aware enough to ask for food or ice. She was borderline delirious and might be in too much pain to type. An anxious, two-mile run back and I opened the door to this annoyed look.

"Didn't you get my text!?" she said while looking me up and down for any hidden hamburgers.

I reminded her that I ran to the gym and had no car but she was not very interested. I told her I could get her one from the cafeteria and she told me they were gross. I stopped for a second because she had not had a burger since we had arrived in Pittsburgh. I asked her if she wanted a burger from the place that just opened by our house in Cincinnati...and she nodded *yes*.

"We're in Pittsburgh."

"Ohhhhhh yeah..."

Her food tray was directly in front of her so I asked her what it was. She had not even lifted the lid to look. "Come on...at least check your tray. You're killin' me."

I could not get too mad at her. She was looking at me with a little poof of hair on the top of her head, unaware of the state that she was in as she apologized. Luckily for both of us, she actually liked the stuffed pepper soup so I did not have to buy anything else. I was not about to jog back to the gym so I guess I was done for the day. My little adventure did take me to the SouthSide Works area and I immediately knew that if we needed an extended stay, that location would be my top choice.

The next morning, PT stopped by early but encountered Rebecca's alter ego, Morning Bec. Between the unexpected visit and the time of day, it was not going to happen. They agreed to come back at 1 p.m. but did not return. As we had our meeting with the transplant social worker, her nurse stopped in and said that she could get Bec into the chair right then but that was her only chance because another patient was checking out. She seemed annoyed when we told her we wanted to finish the transplant discussion with the social worker. She mumbled something about how long she had been doing this and that Becca needed to get up and move. It's a good thing to get somebody with some experience, but if they randomly TELL you they have experience, they are probably insecure.

When she returned to the room, she was still annoyed that Becca had not gotten into the chair and then made some comments about how important that was. I cannot remember the exact words but they came across a bit patronizing and as if Becca was being lazy. I told her that Bec was very motivated for PT and that she had pushed through it on the toughest of days. I also said she needed more notice than someone randomly opening the door and saying now or never, particularly when she was in the middle of something. I continued that she had been working hard and doing this every day for months. I gave her a little attitude because she needed it. Rebecca was willing to work but she needed to be part of the planning process. We had also been waiting to have some of these transplant discussions for months. The last thing Bec needed was somebody insinuating she was lazy, which was no motivation for her—she found it infuriating.

After this great interaction, it was no surprise when the nurse did not accept my offer of help during a transfer to the commode. She actually told me to "skedaddle" as she and another nurse moved her because the room would be "too crowded." I just moved to the corner of the room because I knew Ms. Experience was in too much of a hurry to pause and think this through well.

They moved a few of her lines, but not all of the right ones. When they finally did get her up and turn her, she had lines going every which way with the vent lines wrapped 270 degrees taut behind her back. It was a mess of a failure and the nurse commented how it would be better the next time because they had done it once. Actually, it would have been fine this time if she had listened to someone who had done it hundreds of times, but whatever. Luckily, we never got her again.

We had dozens of nurses over the course of the year. Some were very authoritarian while others were more receptive. Some were motherly while others seemed detached. They shouldered much of the responsibility for her care so as a patient's spouse, it was important to respect this. However, it was on me to ensure that I advocated for both her care and her peace of mind, particularly because she literally could not speak and often could not speak for herself.

To me, one of the most important attributes of a nurse was whether or not he or she could take suggestions. I was cautious of being pushy, but I spent all day every day with this one particular patient and I tried to be an asset. I was good at keeping her calm and knew the better ways to transfer her. Another positive attribute was whether they reviewed her medications with her prior to crushing them and putting them into her feeding tube. For instance, Creon did not crush and would clog the tube so she swallowed that. There was an order in for Senna (a laxative) that had been discontinued but for some reason kept showing back up in the orders. Essentially, it came down to good communication.

I had to watch out for those that would use patronizing tones or scare tactics first. This was more common when Rebecca was at her weakest. At one point, one nurse delivered some bad news about a partially collapsed lung in a way to suggest that it was Rebecca's fault for not doing all she could. She warned that Bec would end up back in the ICU if she was not compliant. That is not how to deliver a diagnosis! I expected them to treat her as an adult with the expectation that she will comply. A collapsed lung is scary enough and does not require any added theatrics. Luckily I was there and was able to point out that she had done all of her PT, then mentioned more than once that the other nurse walked with her when PT could not. Rebecca chimed right in and offered to walk but her nurse backpedaled with some reason why she could not help right then. Of course five minutes later I had crafted this great speech about how much Rebecca had overcome and how this lady's patronizing tone was not appreciated and ineffective. I never got to vocally deliver that speech but it sounded pretty hardcore in my head.

The biggest red flag for me was the experience card. If they responded to any requests with the number of years they were doing the job, it meant one of two things: either they were trying to comfort Rebecca by confirming that she was in good hands, or they themselves were insecure. If they were insecure, the day was going to be a challenge. An insecure nurse would usually not take suggestions well because they "knew better." I found the best approach in many of these situations was to mention that another nurse or therapist had done it a particular way that worked well. I might casually explain how "they" transferred her in a few succinct sentences. They would take it better if I presented it like I had observed one of their colleagues solve this problem rather than as though I had experience or figured out a better way. When they started struggling, it gave them some direction or an "out" to ask me how it was done.

Lesson 27: There's a thin line between telling nurses how to do their job and advocating for a loved one. Be aware of it, but know that you can dig your heels in.

It was reassuring to remember that I always had the ability to "fire" them.

Aside from some stumbling blocks, PT ramped up quickly and Becca was able to walk daily. Her CO_2 levels had improved as well (down from around 100 mEq/L to the low 70s) and we were feeling pretty good. They even removed her arterial line that was set up for frequent blood gases. Everything looked good except her edema that seemed to be creeping back a little each day. Since movement was the best cure for that, we were doing what we could. PT came in to walk her every other day and we were doing our workouts in the room as well. The main challenge was the fact that she was so sleepy. Even though her CO_2 had come down, she was tired all of the time. Two blood transfusions in one week did not help the matter either. I knew that all of this would seem like less of an issue once she was listed.

It was Monday night and I knew the decision was coming on Tuesday. It was like Christmas Eve...I had no chance of sleeping. I would drift off here and there but I was basically staring at the wall. I knew the answer would be *yes*...unless it was *no*. But I could not worry about it being no because there was nothing I could do about that at night. I could only ask for the next steps if that verdict came. But I would not have to ask for those steps because the answer would be *yes*.

If the answer was unequivocally no, we would be out of conventional options. UPMC was our last shot as they tackled the toughest of cases, undaunted by the challenge. In the back of my mind I thought we *could* go to Canada or Mexico maybe, really exploring all of the less conventional options. Besides, we would not have to worry because they already said she looked like a good candidate, right? Of course there was still the committee…ahhhhhhh!

I showed up early with a hope to grab any doctor that came within 50 feet of her room. I first caught the nurse. I asked her when I would find out and who would tell me but she did not know. She seemed to think the meeting was later in the day. When the pulmonologist came around, he said the same thing but added that somebody from the transplant team would be by to tell me the decision. So we waited. Then Bec fell asleep and I waited. As the time ticked by, I texted a few updates, posted online, and otherwise felt amazingly useless.

I decided that the best thing I could do was to focus on the positive. She *would* get accepted and I would need a long-term housing solution. I started my apartment search. I had already checked into a few places that the hospital recommended but once I did the math, a furnished apartment with no lease cost too much.

One option was a place called Family House, which was essentially a hotel with a full kitchen that was set up for reasonably priced, long-term stays near the hospital. Family House was the cheapest and was quite appealing, but they did not take cats. I knew when Bec was out of the hospital and recovering, she would require a LOT of cat time. Another option was a furnished month-to-month rental that quoted me $3,300 a month! Alternatively, nice places in SouthSide Works were going for $1,500 a month. These were unfurnished and required a one-year lease but they would be our own space. Even with a reasonable penalty for early termination that type of place would still cost me less in total.

As I searched and time passed, I was getting more and more anxious. I made the nurse call the doctor several times and he had not heard anything which he said was odd. "Odd" is not good, on this night in particular. Around 9:30, I was told that they would be by in the early morning. All of this waiting just to be told to wait some more…!? I was exhausted and annoyed.

They say during the day before a fight, a new fighter expends most of his energy before he steps into the ring, from nerves. That was exactly how I felt and I still had to go back to the hotel and try to sleep again, knowing that the answer was coming. I went back to the hotel and I tried.

The next morning I saw the doctor outside of the room on the phone. I caught some key words like "cystic" and "transplant" but he stayed just out of earshot. I thought that if the answer was yes, they would already be at the door delivering the great news. When he came to her door, I did not read him as preparing to deliver bad news. He said that the conversation regarding Rebecca was positive, but they were not ready to list her. The way it worked was that some candidates would get a clear *no* right away. Others would get a *yes*. Most would get a *Maybe, how about some more tests?* That was us.

They had a few more tests that they wanted to run. They were looking for an antibody test, a pap smear, another walk, and a repeat of the twenty-four-hour urine test. It could be another four or five days. I bordered on the edge of frustration and appreciation. The longest wait was for the antibody test that required a blood sample. Why did they not take the antibody blood samples earlier? I felt that these were things that could have easily been done concurrently. On the other hand, her urine output was unusually low and she would have probably failed had they not reordered it. We hoped that with some more fluids, she would pass. It was clear that they were doing everything they could for us to qualify, so if it required a bit more waiting then so be it. I had become quite good at waiting even if it was not my favorite skill to utilize.

I had my fingers crossed that nothing new would go wrong; however given enough time, something always went wrong. With her edema increasing and her recent issue with CO_2, there was enough to make me nervous.

They were good at having her walk with some level of frequency but her distances were just not as high or consistent as they had been. We were mostly walking about 130 feet though she had previously achieved 220 feet. Perhaps she was getting weaker but I had to remind myself that they did not require a 500 feet walk. She was not *too* weak.

When Rachel and my mom arrived, they were a bit surprised at how Rebecca looked. She held almost as much edema as in January and she was now disoriented from the ICU delirium. She had become harder to understand when "speaking" and would doze off during sentences. Her lips would be moving fast but were not forming words clearly. I realized that most of my recent updates had included more about the status of the work-up and not very much on the rest of her condition. Perhaps that was because I had hoped it would just pass. I did everything I knew to do which included turning up the lights during the day, playing music, and trying to engage in conversation. The problem was that she was tired all the time now and 'round the clock snoozers did not help her delirium.

At one point, she wanted to tell us something and we struggled to guess what it was. When she began to write it on her dry erase board, she had little success because she was trying to write with the straw from her Boost Breeze. When I handed her the marker, she tried to shove that into her drink. It was a mess.

She settled into one of her naps and we all went for a walk to find a place outside to sit. On a nice park bench, we got to chatting and were just enjoying the weather. In the back of my mind I wondered if Bec was awake. I checked in and her nurse told me that she was still sleeping so we stayed out another forty minutes or so. When we returned, our nurse informed us of an incident and immediately the dread and the guilt rushed back yet again.

Apparently, the connection from the vent slipped off and Rebecca panicked. She was not able to reconnect it herself and her nurse was in another room bagging a patient. I could see it as he was describing the event. First, getting a wave of anxiety and then feeling that escalate as different bells and alarms went off. As her sats dropped, she would have felt out of breath as she struggled to pull in air. Maybe she panicked and hyperventilated again. I could imagine the fear and the helplessness of this once independent woman.

The door was closed and I peeked in to see her completely exhausted. If we had only not taken that last forty minutes to chat, I could have been there to fix it. I had tried a hundred times to show her how to reconnect the tubing if it slipped off but it was always difficult for her. As she always said, she was not very spatial—and with her delirium, it was even harder.

Later that night as we walked out, my mom tried to comfort me with some information that the nurse told her. She said that Rebecca could still breathe but just wasn't getting as much support. I know she was trying to make me feel better and show me that I did not need to be in the room all of the time but it did not change how horrible it was that it happened and that I was not there to help her. I was short with her because I just did not want to talk about it. I did not need a rationalization on why I should not feel guilty because I already knew that rationale. I agreed with the logic but hearing someone else explain it only made me want to poke holes in it. When I saw myself getting frustrated, all I could do was change the subject and pretend that I was over it.

Since turning off the daytime tube feed, all Rebecca needed to do was eat 1,500 calories a day. This had been no problem at the Drake Center and I spent a lot of effort convincing the staff here that she could do that with no problem. I was tracking all of her calories so I could show them how well she would be able to eat. We could order what we wanted and the food was pretty good. After a few days, we developed a routine. The food would arrive, and I would be starving. I would talk it up to Rebecca hoping she would have a go at it right away, so I could get fresh leftovers but she was usually not in the mood. After a nap and a reheat, she would be ready to eat but her few small bites took so long that it would get cold again. I would not let

Bec know that I was counting on it to be my dinner because I wanted her to eat as much as possible instead of just telling me to eat it. When she was finally done, I would scavenge her twice-heated-yet-cold-food that had smelled so good just two hours earlier. I needed a better system and she needed a better appetite.

For a short while, she scraped by with barely enough calories. I was convinced that a mocha latte breve (which I had finally learned to order), a couple of Boosts, and a full-fat yogurt would be the magic ticket. Soon however, she was only taking in about 1,000 calories because she was so sleepy and kept getting bloated. As a last ditch effort to continue her meals, I tried to convince her to eat a yogurt. She shut me down by closing her eyes and repeating that she wanted tube feed, she wanted tube feed. She was depressed and exhausted and no longer wanted to make the effort. Intuitively, I assumed there was something better about eating real food verses merely subsisting on tube feed. It felt like it was more than just a different source of nutrition. I was seeing tube feed as a step back. Going back to tube feed felt like giving up. In the end, I suppose it did not matter how she got her nutrition but I did not want her to give up. Her increasing depression and delirium made it feel like she was slipping away.

Interestingly enough, her delirium was getting worse but I was the one who looked like an idiot. I would try to get her to eat or exercise but she would just close her eyes. Sometimes when I got serious and really called her name she would open them but she would just look past me. I would try to spoon feed her and she would occasionally open up for the food, while somehow simultaneously ignoring me. One night at dinner I must have really been a sight for people near the room. She was hungry and wanted to eat and that was where the battle began.

"Rebecca...Rebecca...you want a bite of soup?" Her eyes were closed yet she was awake. "You liked this soup. You want to try? Here." Closed mouth denial of the spoon and then I get a little soup on her lip. She licks it off while being careful not to open her mouth.

"What about tilapia? It sure smells good! Here, try this bite." The spoon gets halfway in then she closes her mouth and the rest falls on her for me to clean up.

"Do you want milk or Ensure?"…pause…"Do you want milk or Ensure?" One more time: "Do you want milk or ensure? You need some Creon, here you go." She remained firm with her mouth secured in an anti-food position.

"Why don't you take two Creon, here...I'll open the Ensure. Ok, you're going to feel the straw, just a little sip." I was trying to get into a closed garage door. Just imagine a moron talking to a bratty kid. This was soon to become every meal, all day long.

As 6 p.m. on Tuesday night arrived, it was starting to feel like the previous week. I was hoping I would not sit there half the night to receive no news. When the nurse stopped in, I asked again when we might hear something. She said she would page the CF doctor. I started feeding Rebecca her dinner and the nurse walked in saying she had some news. The team had unofficially accepted her and the only thing pending was some additional antibody tests and a dental exam. I was thrilled—unofficially!

I texted the family the good news though I did not yet want to post anything on Facebook. I got something of an acknowledgment from Rebecca but her stomach was bothering her and she could not get comfortable. As she continued to adjust herself, her sats started dropping, her lung pressures were rising, and her blood pressure was through the roof (216/115 mmHg). At this point it was only slightly alarming for me.

Rachel called me just ecstatic. I was too, but it was hard to really enjoy that with Rebecca still so upset. She had kicked a pillow off the bed and tried unsuccessfully to roll to a more comfortable position. Her face was red and she was sweating, even with the fan close to her. There were bells and alarms going off all around us and nurses and RTs were coming into and out of the room. I just wanted Becca to partake in the celebration and to take a moment to reflect. She should enjoy the news that she had gone from the prognosis of a few more days, to maybe a 70 percent chance if they found lungs in time. As I lost hope that she would enjoy the news, my thoughts shifted to just wanting them to drug her so she could get a good night's sleep.

CHAPTER 19

Losing Faith

When I arrived the next morning, Becca looked distressed. She had only taken a few bites of her food and she was sweating. She complained about being bloated and uncomfortable. Her nurse was there asking some questions to see if she was disoriented. Becca knew she was in Pittsburgh, in a hospital, and that it was May 2015 but nothing more than that. As soon as she heard it was the 27th she lit up and wished me a happy birthday. For a brief moment she was there, cheerful and smiling. It had been a while since I had seen this Rebecca. I had not even seen it the night before when we heard that she was close to being listed. Unfortunately, it faded quickly as the nurse left and she struggled to get comfortable. Before long it dropped to a new low.

"I can't do this anymore. I'm done." I read from her lips. "I can't do this anymore. I'm done." She repeated over and over. She looked so exhausted.

Knowing but not wanting to know, I asked "What can't you do?"

"I can't do this. I want to go."

"Where do you want to go?"

"I want to go home. I'm done. I'm done. This is too hard."

"I know it's hard, baby, but we need the vent, and the vent is here. Soon you'll be listed and we'll be waiting for new lungs to arrive. Imagine how much better things will be with your new lungs. We'll sit outside with a nice cup of coffee, go hiking...it'll be so much better, right?"

She smirked slightly and agreed that it would be nice. I told her my birthday gift would be her getting listed and her birthday gift (in eleven days) would be new lungs. She liked that.

She fell into a deep sleep and when PT came in to walk her, she wanted nothing to do with it. She was just going to lay there and sleep but we talked her into getting into the chair. I kept throwing it out to her that if she stood up to get in the chair that maybe she could take a few steps...whatever she was up for.

As we started to manage her various lines and move her pillows, the PT and RT had given up on it. Then, not more than a minute into the transfer, she agreed to walk. I was surprised and so happy. This is exactly what we needed, both to show the doctors and to keep her muscles moving. We lined her up and she took off like a shot with that walker. She went all the way to the doors at the end of the hall where she normally stopped, and just kept going. Even one of the other patients cheered her on from her room as Rebecca went by. She totaled 250 feet that day which was the most she had done since coming to Pittsburgh.

I was genuinely shocked that day and I was the most proud of her I had ever been. She had come from such a low place that morning to do so well that afternoon. I could see it in her eyes; she came alive for that moment. Afterward, she looked better even though she was tired. I could see that she had a mood shift in a positive direction, but most of all, I could see that she had a sense of accomplishment. It was one of those battles that we needed to win.

Becca suffered through a lot of ups and downs. Despite her success with physical therapy, her spirits were creeping progressively lower and she was becoming disoriented more frequently. It was a bad combination. The next day, she was more restless than I had ever seen her. She could not decide whether she wanted to stay in the bed or get in the chair. During the quiz from the nurse, she said it was 2010 (instead of 2015). She could not speak clearly or focus well either.

I would start to work through my to-do list but every two minutes I would hear her tapping on the bed, requiring my attention. When she spoke, it was so hard to understand. The dry erase board did not help because she could no longer write legibly. I finally got from her that she wanted pain meds. I asked if she was in a lot of pain or just wanted some help sleeping. It was the latter of the two. At two in the afternoon, the last thing we needed was something to help her sleep! I explained as I did so many times before that we wanted her to be awake as much as possible during the day. It would help with the delirium, it would help her sleep at night, and we would be able to visit a little more because I would not be there at night.

There was little reasoning with her in this state. When she finally did get in her chair, she was back and forth between reclining and sitting up. She would ask for the nurse but then could not remember what she wanted. She said she was perpetually exhausted. She reached a level of restlessness that was new and dangerous. She would make these large, unexpected movements with her upper body and it was causing her to pop off the vent more frequently. It was not long before she had stood up on her own. All of her pillows and blankets fell to the floor and her trach tubes were just dangling there. She just about gave me a heart attack.

She also had a lot to say. I could not decipher it all but she simply looked sad. She made a face like she was going to cry but did not have the energy. When she thought she heard the doctor outside, she perked up and looked around like she was on a mission. From her lips I read the worst thing I could imagine: "Tell the doctor I quit!" she said. "Tell the doctor I quit! Tell the doctor I quit! Tell the doctor I quit! Tell the doctor I quit!"

She just repeated it over and over. Her lips were mouthing those words, while her eyes closed....closed to any feedback because she did not want to listen. Shaking her head back and forth, she just sat there repeating. "Tell the doctor I quit!" Here we were, so close to getting listed after such a tough road, almost at a point where her chance of surviving the next year would shift from "unlikely" to "about 70 percent" and she wanted to quit. I felt like I had to whisper my response because I did not want anybody knowing what she was saying. This was the second time she was talking along these lines and she was more adamant. What if she said this to the wrong person? How could they list someone who had given up!? I did not feel it was being suicidal but if they categorized it as such, would our chances fall apart?

Whatever I said could not be grand enough to communicate the importance of her words at that moment. I could not be enlightening enough to shift her focus to the fragile nature of the situation. All I could do was remind her of how far she had come, and how she was so close to something better. Tenacious B had inspired so many, maybe she could channel that for a little bit longer.

I told her how good she would feel and all of the things she would be able to do again. I even asked her what she would want me to do if I were in that situation. I was searching for anything that worked. I never got a real response. I hugged her around all of the tubes and wires, and put my cheek to hers. "I love you, baby. I don't want to lose you."

Her eyes were closed through all of this. It was her only way of escaping. No matter what I tried, it continued. She just kept shaking her head asking me to "Go tell the doctors. Tell them I quit."

As quickly as that bad turn in the conversation, she faded off to sleep. I was left with this new burden, one that she had hinted at previously but never said so boldly and so defiantly. As I sat with my thoughts, the pre-transplant coordinator walked in. It was the worst timing imaginable. I put on my happy face and let her wake Rebecca. She awoke calm and pleasant but all I could wonder was how she would respond. If she started spouting the same things she was before, we were in trouble.

We got through most of the discussion with no hiccups until she asked us if we had questions. Rebecca, of course, had questions. I could not tell exactly what she said but it looked hauntingly similar to what she had been saying: "I want to quit."

In this state, she was harder to read, particularly for people that were not used to her, and the coordinator could not understand what she was saying. I felt a rush of adrenaline kick in as I tried to think of how to avoid any bad turns. I acted confused "What...you want to eat? What do you want to eat?" As she responded, she spoke faster and became even harder to read. At this point, neither of us were able to discern what she was saying. I picked out another two words that looked like "tube feed" and I had sold it. That was not the coordinator's department and we temporarily dodged another bullet.

I sat there thinking, "You're killing me, Rebecca... killing me." But I had done what I needed to do. She could still decide to quit but she should not decide rashly or on a whim, particularly when she was not in her right mind. A statement like that might have to go into her medical record and work against her. She had every right to change her mind but this was not the way.

People could debate about her state of mind and whether she could make her own decisions, they could debate whether or not I had the right to do what I did, but I did it. After she drifted back to sleep, I jogged to the SouthSide to arrange things for our apartment. I thought I had left her in a good place but she popped off her vent. By the time they had made it to Rebecca, her sats were in the 50s. When I called to check in, they explained the incident. Her movements were getting larger and more reckless. She was so uncomfortable that she must have leaned forward without regard to her trach, causing the vent tubes to dislodge again.

When I returned, she told me that Jessica was crying. Had her sister really called earlier or was it part of the delirium? Either way, she wanted to discuss it. I asked her when they had spoken and Bec said, "Before."

"Before what...?"

"...before I was dying."

As long as it had been, she could still say things that hit me right in the chest. That was how she explained her incident. I imagined her in a silent panic with no voice to call for help as she gasped for air hearing all of the bells and alarms going off all around her. I felt like I could never leave the room. I was out doing errands while she was terrified, unable to breathe, thinking she was dying alone in a strange hospital room.

As the day went on, her spirits got even worse. She was in and out of sleep and I would hear her tap for my attention over and over again but understood less and less of what she was saying. The only thing I knew was the urgency in her eyes. She had started to feel her trach and try to move it, seemingly to a more comfortable position. All of a sudden I saw her face melt into a cry as she was holding on to this thing that was both keeping her alive, and imprisoning her in her chair. I put my face to hers and told her I loved her.

She said what looked like, "I want to die." She said it over and over shaking her head from side to side. I could not bring myself to confirm what she was saying and I don't think I would have understood the answer if I did. All I knew was that time was running out and she needed something big to change her state of mind.

Maybe if Jessica came out again it might lift her spirits. She had held off because Becca was not listed yet so we wanted to be sure of the listing before she flew out. In a few moments, the priority shifted to improving Rebecca's spirits. I called Jessica and told her that Rebecca needed her immediately. I gave her a partial explanation of the events that had led to the call and asked her to trust me. This was the time to come. It was my best move because Jessica was my ace in the hole. Pete had her back and helped with the travel costs so we would make it happen. This HAD to help.

Lesson 28: Do not hesitate to ask for help.

The apartment situation was a whole 'nother headache. I had looked into a few local places that rented furnished apartments by the day to people in our situation. The cheapest option came out to about $1,850 per month. The rooms were so-so and had some nice common areas but they did not allow cats. Unfortunately Becca would want her cats at her side while she was recovering, they were a good pick-me-up.

The next best option was $3,500 per month and we could bring our cats if they passed the "pet interview." For this price I could cryogenically freeze her cats and not have to deal with the kitty litter. I finally decided on a single bedroom unfurnished apartment for $1,800 that included parking. It would be the least expensive option, even considering a penalty to break the lease and the cost of a little furniture.

I was jogging down to L.A. Fitness in the SouthSide Works

area to exercise and found I really liked the area. It had fancy shops, coffee houses with outdoor seating areas, restaurants, and bakeries. All of this was right up Bec's alley; she would love it! I focused my search on that location and found a few nice options. I figured if I leveraged my sob story, somebody might be willing to allow a six-month lease. I tried this brilliant approach with one apartment and the landlord agreed to it on the spot. Just before I left to meet her the next day, she called and said that her husband had vetoed that plan and they would not do a six-month lease. Though I was still interested in seeing the place, suddenly the apartment would be unavailable for another month because her tenant had asked to extend. I was not sure how much of that was true but it was clear that I had scared her away.

My new approach had to be, "It is *probably* a year...but out of curiosity...what is the cancellation policy *if* something comes up?" The next place had a great cancellation policy...for them. I would have to give two months' notice but would be responsible for paying the rent until they leased it to someone else. I called one place after the next and very few had something available for June. In fact, the only place that had availability, elevators, and a clear cancelation policy was actually the nicest.

The only problem was that they did not allow pets. Surely that did not apply to *our* cats, Paul and Priscilla. I felt that there was an unspoken exception that as long as I hid them, their foolish rules did not apply to us. Yep, this place was meant to be. I filled out the application and set a move-in date that was soon enough to get me out of the hotel but allowed enough time to confirm that she was listed. By this time we were only waiting on one more antibody test, the results of which they estimated would be in within twenty-four to forty-eight hours.

Unfortunately, it took closer to a week. Every day we thought we would get our answer and every day we heard nothing. The day had come to sign the lease and she was not yet listed. I had a knot in my stomach because I knew I was taking a risk. I just had this need to move forward. This was the only place with availability in June and an apartment was a huge cost savings over staying at the hotel. Besides, the staff discussed her listing as almost a foregone conclusion and we just needed that one last test.

The day I went to sign the lease, she was still not listed and I stood in my new empty apartment calling the hospital as a last ditch effort for results while I put off signing. I was actually able to postpone signing for a few more days but eventually they needed it and I signed a one-year lease without confirmation that Rebecca was going to be listed. I was really more concerned that Rebecca was not going to survive until the transplant. By signing that lease, I told myself that I was betting on Rebecca's future, and that felt good...albeit dumb.

I returned to the hospital to see that the focus had shifted from waiting for lab results to rising CO_2 levels. I hoped that the standard airway clearance would work...percussive therapy, breathing treatments, suction, and time.

As soon as the nurse asked me if the doctor had explained the plan if this did not work, I knew this was different. The look on her face made it clear that this was serious. If her CO_2 did not drop and her pH did not rise, they were planning to put Bec on ECMO (extracorporeal membrane oxygenation). This meant that they were going to cycle her blood through a machine that would oxygenate it and remove the carbon dioxide. She would likely be on this for the entire time she waited for the transplant. I did not know much about this but I knew it was a big deal. One doctor had told me that once she was on ECMO, the clock would start and she could survive for roughly two weeks. Her lungs would still be ventilated to slow the degradation. This was basically done to bridge the gap to transplant.

The problem with hearing the backup plan late at night was that no one was there to answer the questions that I did not want to ask. So I was left with hoping and praying that this issue cleared up. The plan was to do a chest X-ray then aggressive airway clearance. This included The Vest (to be used with Rebecca positioned at several different angles) as well as lavage. She was so exhausted they did not believe she could sit up at the edge of the bed without falling asleep and falling off. So I sat there beside her to hold her up, the whole time afraid of what was coming yet trying to remain optimistic for both of us. I could hear a great deal of concern in the voices of her caregivers, which confirmed my fears.

When the therapy was done and the initial results came back, her numbers had improved slightly. ECMO was not going to happen that night and an aggressive treatment plan was set up for airway clearance every two hours. By midnight, I felt comfortable enough to leave.

Over the next two days, her CO_2 remained high but the

doctors commented how surprising it was that she was tolerating it. We hoped that getting up and walking would mobilize some of the secretions and we would start seeing improvements with suctioning.

My view for the next walk was from behind the chair I was pushing and it was tough to watch. She took off like a shot. Well...maybe not a shot but fast for somebody using a walker. I started to feel optimistic as she got out of the door and into the hallway. But then she stopped. We were only a few steps in and she stopped. Then she did something she had never done before — she leaned against the wall. It appeared that we were done with the walk after just a few steps. I wanted so badly for her to push off and keep moving. I had never wished more powerfully that I could take her place.

She stood there, leaning against the wall for probably twenty seconds. I knew she was determined to go farther than her weakened body would allow. As she pushed off, her knees buckled and I watched from behind as she crumbled toward the ground. The nurse caught her as she collapsed while I stood there watching my hopes fall in front of me, wondering if the listing and new lungs would come in time. Even if they did, how much damage had her body already experienced? Thinking about what could be going through her mind filled me with empathy. She was working so hard and her body was just giving out on her.

I did not know how I was going to leave her to get our things from Cincinnati but at some point it would be necessary. It felt selfish because I knew I could just stay in Pittsburgh and sleep on the air mattress in our new apartment. What I did not want to admit was that I did not know if she would survive long enough to require the trip. Was this all just a stupid waste of time? I knew I should not think like that but I was questioning my own intelligence for committing to a twelve-month lease.

I now had an apartment; I was ready to get some of my things, so I felt like it was now or never. The best case scenario would be her getting listed over the next couple of days and I definitely would not want to leave after that. I could just imagine getting "the call" but being four and a half hours away and in the middle of packing. There would never be a perfect time. I also wanted to go because it was simply being optimistic. By going, I was betting that Rebecca would get listed, transplanted, and be in Pittsburgh for a while.

Always ready to help, our friend Meg came up to stay with Rebecca so that I could head home. Then after she drove all the way up from South Carolina, I became uncertain whether or not I should go. I was, however, looking forward to having a couch and real bed and I knew that she was in good hands with Meg.

We sat there that Sunday morning looking at Rebecca and knowing her blood gases had not improved. My plan switched back and forth between getting the rental car and waiting. On one hand, I had not been away from Rebecca for twenty-four hours since this had started and now she was sicker than she had been in a while. On the other hand, I would not have someone there to stay with Rebecca if I waited any longer. My dad was meeting me at my house and even though he could stay there for a few days, I wanted to get the move over with.

I finally decided to go and I was on a mission. I was concerned because things were getting worse with Rebecca so I had to go and get back as quickly as possible. It was only four and a half hours but it seemed like an eternity. I came through my door ready to go. I had this list that I had been developing for a couple of weeks and I knew everything I needed. I got it together and packed it in record time while I waited for my dad to arrive. I packed late and woke early. I made it to the bank, the rental car return, the DMV, and a neighbor's to buy another couch. We packed up the SUV and pickup in the rain, then secured a tarp over the top.

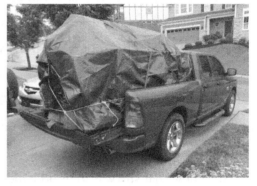

We got on the road around 3 p.m., later than I would have liked but still not too bad. As we drove, a call came in from Pennsylvania. Was it Pittsburgh? Had something horrible happened? Had she finally received the last test results and was listed?

It turned out to be Aetna. The lady told me that the insurance company had approved her transplant. It was good news, but did not really make sense. As far as I knew, we were still waiting for the last antibody test to return. She said that Rebecca was listed but I was not quite sure if they were getting it right. I assumed I would get the first call but maybe I had a pending call from the hospital confirming her listing. What amazing, confusing news! Perhaps they were the loose-lipped neighbor who ruined the surprise party.

Regardless of the rain and distance we still had to travel, the anxiety started to melt away. I had this sense that it was all going to be okay, as I looked forward to a call from the hospital. A couple of hours into the ride, my friend Meg called. As soon as she said that she was there with the doctors I KNEW they were calling to tell me that Rebecca was listed. I waited with a smile as she led up to it. Then, they dropped the bomb. Becca's rising CO_2 levels would necessitate putting her on ECMO. It was like a sucker punch and it completely took me off guard.

I rambled through my questions knowing the whole time that I would agree to it. They did not take this lightly and her CF doctor told me that he would only consider it as a last resort. The concern was that once she was on it, she would only be able to survive for about two weeks. This was terrifying. She was not even listed yet and now she had roughly two weeks to get listed AND be lucky enough to get matching donor lungs. I suddenly felt so far away and regretted not being there for it. The only consolation was that because of her elevated CO_2 levels and delirium she was not totally "with it" and did not fully understand what was going on.

I continued cruising along ten miles below the speed limit, watching my dad's truck in the rearview, and going out of my mind. All I wanted to do was take-off and tell my dad to meet me there but I knew we would not be allowed in to see her by the time I arrived so there was no point. We headed to the apartment to unload and I unpacked and organized until about 2:30 in the morning. I would soon be spending a lot of time in the hospital and would have little opportunity to get this done later.

We arrived early to find large red tubes connected to Rebecca. I quickly learned that it was not actually the tubes that were red, it was the blood filling them, routing their way to and from the ECMO machine. She looked so vulnerable and helpless. All I could think was that the ticking clock had started. I had a hard time looking at her as she slept there. It was a lot like in January when she was first intubated. There was all of this new equipment that was intimidating and signified a decline in Rebecca's overall condition. There was even a person called a perfusionist tasked with monitoring her ECMO machine at all times.

These tubes connected to veins in her neck and groin and the risk of kinking these large catheters was high. She wore a headband to protect the neck catheter from excessive movement and could not turn her head more than a few degrees. The groin catheter was stitched to her right leg at five different spots and she could not bend it for fear of kinking or pulling the catheter. After months of being uncomfortable in her bed, her situation had somehow worsened. A few inches here and a few degrees there was her full range of motion. It required four people just to get her into a recliner. If her spirits were low before, I worried the next two weeks of this would destroy them.

This setup was not what I was expecting. They had planned to do an Avalon arrangement which would have had both the input and output in her neck allowing her to move more freely. With it, she could have stood and even walked. I asked why they used this arrangement knowing that I would probably not like the answer. During transportation to the procedure, Rebecca experienced a major issue.

She desatted and then decompensated, which was kind of a general term meaning that one of her systems had stopped functioning properly. In her case, it was cardiac decompensation, a fast and dangerous drop of her heart rate. They needed to perform the procedure emergently and had no time to do the Avalon arrangement.

They said that they could potentially change her to the Avalon style but we would have to wait since she would be recovering from that trauma for a few days. The more I heard about it the less likely it sounded, particularly because the required flow rate of her blood through the ECMO machine was too high for the Avalon and she was too weak.

We had attributed her prolonged survival on the ventilator to all of her physical therapy. Suddenly, it was no longer an option during the most critical time of her care. I worried that the lack of movement would take her to the shorter side of those two weeks. She remained on a ventilator as well even though the ECMO machine was doing much of the work to oxygenate her blood and remove the CO_2. The point was to keep her lungs moving and working even if they were not accomplishing much.

The transplant doctor stopped in and said that the last antibody test was still not back yet. This particular antibody test was supposed to take twenty-four to forty-eight hours to come back and we had now been waiting for over a week. To top it off, they had redrawn blood for the test the day before and we had no idea what was going on with it. I asked him about it and he seemed to think there may have been some mistake or something missed but really did not have any answers. I pressed him pretty hard about what we could do to expedite and he said he would call the lab and try to get an answer that night. I asked if we could take more blood and send them out to several labs simultaneously or do something else to ensure an expedited answer. He told me they would do whatever they could to get an answer that day. Since she was now on ECMO, every day we waited could be the difference between life and death.

The hours passed and Becca lay there and slept. She looked terrible. Despite the ventilator and ECMO machine, her O_2 sats were not stellar as they floated around in the low 90s. I sat there for a long time looking at the area behind her bed because it was too hard to look at her directly. Meanwhile, Rebecca wandered in and out of consciousness looking as down as I had ever seen her.

I was sitting there with my father when my phone rang; it was Rachel. I recapped the recent string of events, while I tried to stay positive especially since I was talking in front of Rebecca. As we spoke, I could see Rebecca appeared increasingly distressed. She was trying to say something to me so I got closer to see what she was saying. My heart sank when I realized she was saying the last thing I ever wanted to hear.

"I want you to kill me."

I paused, I still had the phone to my ear and my sister was talking about one of the fundraisers.

"I want you to kill me."

I told my sister I had to go and handed the phone to my father.

"I want you to kill me. I know you can do it." She had this look of determined desperation. I told her how close we were to getting approved and that new lungs would be just around the corner.

"I want to die, Die, DIE!" she said in defiance. I had no high CO_2 levels to blame this day while I scrambled for a response. She looked into my eyes, "I am in hell."

"In hell you would not have people who loved you sitting by your side." To that she nodded with this small movement which was all that her cannula would allow.

All I could do was empathize with her and her pain and try to refocus her on a future with new lungs. "I KNOW it's been a long year and that you feel awful right now. But we are so close to a transplant that we could be listed today and could get lungs within a week. All of the pain and frustration you're dealing with now will be resolved with new lungs. All of these IVs and ECMO will go away, the vent will go away, you'll be able to get stronger and you'll have more energy! I've found this great little place for us not far from the hospital. It has a ton of little coffee houses we can walk to and just sit outside. The area has tons of shops and there's a bakery downstairs that will even deliver to our room..."

I went on and on like a desperate man trying to not sound desperate. She calmed down slightly but nothing could take that vision from my mind. Her face was adamant and defiant while pained and afraid. The silent surrender that I had feared for the past week had finally arrived. This was no longer a hint open to interpretation...this was the clear, brutal reality of her wishes. There was nothing I could say or do to change her state of mind.

As I sat in the aftermath of our discussion, I felt hopeless. Bec was not listed, she had given up hope, the ECMO timeline had begun, and she was as sick as I had ever seen her. Was I wrong for continuing to push her toward this transplant? If her wishes had changed and her mind was no longer in a fog, was I wrong to say nothing while she was asking me to speak for her? Was I just torturing this poor woman who had already been through so much?

What could I even do? Could I have them take her off the machine and watch her crash? I could not even ask that question while we still had hope. All of this self-doubt was swirling around but I kept doing the one thing that felt right, imagining our goal. It was an impossible situation and though I was trying my hardest, it did not feel like I was succeeding at keeping her spirits up. My approach had been to try to get her to see things from a certain perspective. The best way I could do that was to try to focus her thoughts on this one possible future. I described our ideal future in detail, helping her to picture the things she loved. With Rebecca, it could not be unrealistic, and there had to be a goal. Spending a nice day outside at a coffee shop, going for a walk, relaxing on our deck on a Saturday…these could all happen after a transplant.

I tried to pull her into the vision and ask her about what she was looking forward to most. I gave her simple examples like watching a movie on the couch or going for a hike. I needed for her to focus on a life that would be better than the present. It was not going to solve her problems but I just needed her to fight a little longer. I had no delusion that my little pep talk would change her mindset, but I hoped to influence it slightly. Like a weak pain medication, maybe it could take the edge off. Those moments of optimism are not wasted; they hold the value of keeping you going.

I knew it was not nearly enough but I was not in control of her mind or her emotions. *She* was fighting this battle and was the only one who could win it. All I could do was remind her of what success looked like, what it felt like.

Lesson 29: The risk of being too hopeful then getting let down is a better option than expecting something miserable from the start.

As I sat there with all of these thoughts going through my head, my phone rang. It was the transplant coordinator. She wanted to confirm if I was told that Rebecca was officially listed. Wait…what!?! REBECCA WAS OFFICIALLY LISTED!!!

"REBECCA'S LISTED??" I said aloud looking at her to see her response. "That's FANTASTIC!"

As the voice on the phone continued, I watched as hope returned to Rebecca's eyes. I knew it would take time to fully sink in but she had a reason to keep fighting. This *could* happen.

She told me her LAS was 91.2 but brought it out to four decimal places, probably because it was one of the highest scores she had ever seen. I asked her where that put Rebecca on the transplant list. After what felt like an eternity, but was probably closer to forty seconds, she told me that there was no one listed higher than her in the region. She was in the number one position! This was so incredibly awesome. After jumping through so many hurdles, we only had one left: finding a donor.

Rebecca never again gave up hope. She never again told me she wanted to quit and she never again said she wanted to die.

A probable listing would not do the job of convincing her that she had a chance, she required an official listing. It was not some amazing speech that inspired her to live. I had given her a bunch of decent pep talks that hopefully inspired her to push a little longer. Little victories add up and much like ECMO, they bridged the gap.

Lesson 30: If you feel like you're losing, keep fighting. You never know when something as simple as a single call can change everything.

My dad was there to hear the news and I immediately texted it out to the rest of the family and then some close friends. I posted it on her Facebook page, short and sweet (just like Bec)...

> **June 2, 2015: Facebook Post:**
> *Listed and sitting in the #1 spot!*

This was thrilling. All we needed to do was wait. Well, wait and survive...but we were down to the last hurdle and the next lungs that became available were hers!

The next day we arrived to see Rebecca in an improved but contemplative mood. I attributed this to a combination of learning that she was listed and becoming more accustomed to her new situation. As I sat next to her, she looked at me concerned. She told me, "I don't want you to forget who I am."

"I know exactly who you are."

"I don't want you to forget who I am outside of this!" she clarified.

"I could never forget," I told her.

It was less about the words that were said and more about the connection we had. In that moment, we both just understood each other. She was a fighter and had been facing down this expected loss for half of a year...her whole life, in a sense. Everyone has moments of weakness, but what mattered was her lifetime of strength. I could never forget her fighting spirit.

CHAPTER 20

The Gathering

After the most recent decline and listing, her mother called for help in planning her visit. It was much better timing than during the evaluation. She informed me that she was coming out and asked for some details to help her nail down her itinerary. If she did not need any info from me I was sure she would have just shown up.

I sent her a text containing all of the best deals for accommodations in the area. I did not think she knew I had an apartment yet but I was not going to offer that she stay there. My dad was there with me and we had a pretty good situation with just the two of us. He was a huge support and drama free.

She arranged to stay at the Family House. Her flight arrived late so she asked me to get her keys for her, which I did. Jessica had planned to arrive a day later and stay with Brenda.

It felt good not to be at home where I would have felt responsible to be a better host. At this point, I was just feeling frustrated with Brenda. Her fundraiser had not happened (with COTA or without). Rebecca had been in the hospital for over 150 days and Brenda had not sent a single card even though I had told everyone that they meant so much to Rebecca. I only hoped that Bec would get something positive out of this visit. After seeing her in this state, maybe Brenda would spend less time on her phone and more time trying to make Rebecca feel better.

I was looking forward to a little gym time because someone would be there to tend to Rebecca's hamburger needs "from with when aldo" while I was gone. After a particularly hard month, I decided to enjoy the benefits of having more support there.

Suddenly, there were four of us there. Jessica and I would do our best to tend to Becca's wants and needs...feeding, hair brushing, shaving, nail clipping. Brenda mostly focused on her phone randomly chatting with Bec and Jess. My dad spent much of his time in the waiting room simply because the CTICU room was small. He would stop in every few hours to check on things. He would chat for a while and ask Rebecca how she was doing then offer her a foot massage which she would promptly accept.

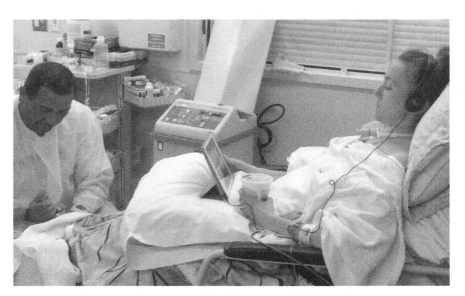

Outside of the room, he focused primarily on keeping his head forward, so he would not snore as he dozed in the recliner. This arrangement worked fairly well and there were no battles for time in the room.

As we all sat there, her sats were bordering on the low 90s, Bec looked fine though her levels should have been much higher with all of the support she was receiving. They told us that her lungs were barely doing anything. Slowly her numbers were creeping down and I could see her nurse and RT had noticed. They came in, bumped her O_2, and tried to suction. Nothing was changing the trend as her sats continued to tick down into the low 80s. The nurse was clearly worried now as she called for the doctor with increasing urgency.

Jessica, Brenda, and I moved just outside the room to be out of the way. Now and again, I would try to say something encouraging to Rebecca as she sat there alert while the staff rushed around her. Jessica and Brenda huddled closer to me as we all stood there nervously waiting for her numbers to improve. By this point, the nurse was visibly upset calling again for the doctor. They started to bag her and it looked like her sats had leveled off.

I put my arm around her sister and mom as we peered around the corner hoping nobody would ask us to leave. Despite our issues, I empathized with both of them, having to see someone they love going through this. The importance of receiving these new lungs quickly was brutally apparent!

The attending physician arrived. Calmly and with confidence he said to give her some sedation to keep her adrenaline down, then to give her more blood to get her H&H (hemoglobin and hematocrit) to the right level. Hemoglobin is critical because it carries oxygen in the blood and the process of being on ECMO often reduces hemoglobin levels. The doctor's calm, confident demeanor served as a comfort to us all. We watched as her sats started to rise slowly...very slowly. Even with the support of ECMO while being bagged, her numbers were slow to rise. This was not my first time witnessing something like this but it was still not easy. I knew it was a tough first day for the ladies but they were able to keep calm. Standing together, we all watched as her sats climbed.

As we moved into the next days, Becca seemed to stabilize a bit. Her health and mood started to improve. Surprisingly enough, the mood started first. About two days after starting on ECMO, her secretions started to get really bloody. They said it might not be anything but still switched to a new, softer suction tube in case there was some suction trauma. Most likely, it was due to the high amounts of heparin they were giving her to keep her from clotting while on ECMO. Though not a major concern, it was unnerving to see all of that blood come out during suctioning. In addition to that, her secretions had actually reduced which seemed unusual. They did a bronch to see if the secretions were collecting anywhere but it came out clean. At this point, my professional medical opinion was that her lungs just kind of sucked.

Desatting instances became the new norm. She would reach the low 80s and it would take a while to come back up. It was unnerving because she was now on ECMO along with a high level of support from the vent so we had little left in the bag of tricks to draw from if things got worse. When an episode did occur, they would bag her or use the vent to "recruit" her. The higher pressures would open up the air sacs. Recruiting on the vent worked better because they never had to disconnect her and it seemed to work more rapidly.

As the frequency increased, both the staff and our little group grew less alerted by each instance. Even Rebecca had come to accept that her numbers may drop with some frequency and it did not seem to bring her as much anxiety. This had become the new norm and part of the daily routine. At shift change they would explain it as something she "does"...kind of like snoring.

During each shift, the nurse would ask Bec a series of questions to confirm her state of mind, one of which was the date. She would understandably get this wrong, but afterwards they would correct her. One morning they told her it was June 3rd, and without a second's pause, Bec said with certainty, "I've been here for thirty days." She had not been, but her incredible confidence made me stop and do the math. Though her CO_2 level had come down quickly after starting ECMO, it took a few days for her delirium to dissipate. The next day, when her new nurse told her it was June 4th, she immediately responded, "I've been here for forty-five days." The nurse was impressed with her quick math.

At the same time, it was nice having the girls there to be with Rebecca because it made my gym time a little less guilt-ridden. Bec had company more of the time which was good because she got depressed when she was alone. While my dad spent much of his time in the waiting room, listening to stories from other families, we got to hear a lot of the action first hand. It is bad form to look or listen in on other patients but it was hard not to overhear from a few feet away with only curtains separating everyone.

A gentleman we'll call Fred had a room across from us. We could not help but hear the nurse speaking loudly to him. "FRED! CAN YOU HEAR ME, FRED? SQUEEZE MY HAND IF YOU CAN HEAR ME, FRED! CAN YOU HEAR ME, FRED?"

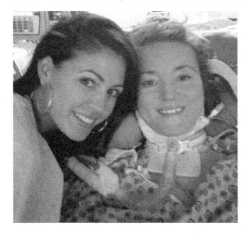

Jessica and I looked at each other and chuckled a little. Of course, we had sympathy for everyone on that floor but there was something kind of funny about this. It was probably how hard the nurse was working and the fact that she used his name in every sentence.

"FRED! SQUEEZE MY HAND, FRED. SQUEEZE MY HAND, FRED..."

While this went on, Jessica and I determined that Fred was Rebecca's favorite neighbor. We envisioned that once she got her lungs, her first stop would be to go visit Fred. "Hey, Fred, LET'S GO!" She would yell to him from her wheelchair. He would hop into his and they would go racing through the hospital halls together. Fred was a little slower than Bec but she would encourage him. "Come on Fred, KEEP IT UP!" Fred would enjoy Bec's positive attitude and the two would become best of friends.

"YOU CAN DO IT, FRED!" she would say. Fred would smile and do his best to pick up the pace. We were not 100 percent sure that this friendship would happen but it seemed like a logical recovery scenario. The whole fabrication was a loopy distraction, but it reflected the mood of light hearted humor we tried to maintain while sitting in this dark hospital room day in and day out.

Since getting listed, Rebecca had found new strength. She had her game face on while dealing with bad news, percussion treatments, and severely limited movement. She was quiet but maintained this survival attitude as she tackled each discussion and new medical reality. She spent a lot of time listening to relaxation sounds with some new noise cancelling headphones. I signed up for an audio book app and she listened to a third of a chapter, once. Focusing on anything but the current situation was essential. Both the loopy fantasy of her friend Fred and the intended effects of Rebecca's calming sounds contributed to one key aspect, the mood. We could not control the bad news, the medical results, or even what we heard around us, but we could do our best to maintain a lighter mood. At times it was hard but I found it worth the effort. Rebecca could either sit in a room surrounded by grimacing faces or surrounded by smiles. My gut told me which option was better.

Lesson 31: Be aware of the mood and try to affect it in a positive way.

On June 7th, Rebecca's thirty-eighth birthday arrived. I stopped at the bakery below my apartment to get her a slice of cake. She had passed her swallow test but the doctors had not approved her to eat because they were still concerned with aspiration. One way or another she was going to get some cake for her birthday even if I had to sneak it to her.

I arrived and my first question was whether the doctor would reconsider her eating. I told the nurse that it was a hard-fought birthday and she needs to celebrate it. Even if we could only get a few bites, she earned this. They heard my argument and said they would consider it. A few minutes later, the doctor came by and said he would approve it, but she must take tiny bites. This was only pleasure eating so we had to keep the total amount to a minimum. I listened with a super serious, contemplative expression on my face. Then I thanked him and it was cake-eating time!

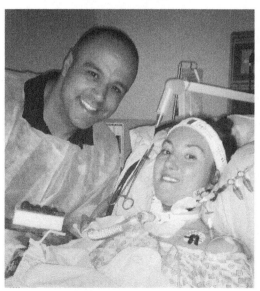

I did make sure I watched the bite size as I fed it to her. I was so happy we could make this happen and she really enjoyed it. We only got about one-fifth of the way through that piece of cheesecake but I got a rare smile that made all of the effort totally worth it.

June 7, 2015 Facebook post

The team here made up a sign for Rebecca's birthday. I also used it to leverage for re-approval to eat some food. "Come on man…you can't deny her birthday cake on a very hard earned birthday!"

Worked like a charm.

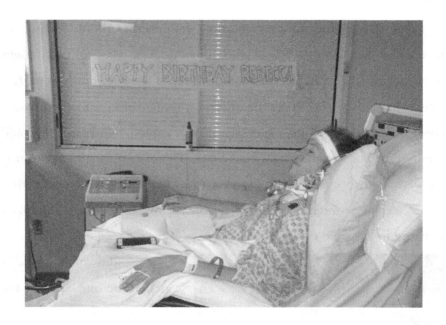

After a morning of shopping, the girls walked in with some gifts for Becca's birthday. Brenda had finally brought her a card even if it was not the get well card she had looked for during the past six months. In fact, she actually handed her a small bag with twenty-two birthday cards in it…

"One for each day," she said as I looked at them confused.

Maybe she meant each birthday and they were supposed to cover her through her fifty-ninth. I would need to watch carefully and see how well it worked because I might have found the golden ticket to never missing an anniversary. "Of course I remembered dear, you know I got you that card twelve years ago! I signed it and everything. Honestly, I'll be hurt if you lost it."

Bec's spirits swung a bit downward as the next days passed. In our heads, we knew she was on the list but it felt like nothing was happening. The routine did not change as we were back and forth every day just hoping for the call. With Bec a little low, I would talk her through the good that was coming more and more frequently.

"How nice will it be when you get out of the surgery and no longer have all of these ECMO tubes? Then you'll only have the trach for a few more days after that. It will be great to roll over in the bed with nobody watching your lines. They'll have you standing and walking again pretty quickly. Remember how good that felt? It won't be long before you're free to walk over to the cafeteria and get some food. The next thing you know, we'll be walking right on home. I can put on an action movie that you have no interest in and you can sleep on me while I play with your hair. We can walk over to one of the coffee shops nearby. There must be a half dozen of them around. You can sit outside and sip your coffee in the sun. It only gets better from here. You know that, right?"

She would look at me in a way that was clear she was listening and maybe imagining. This time, I knew it helped.

Lesson 32: To stay motivated, maintain a vision of the future you want and try to imagine living it.

CHAPTER 21

Apocalypse Soon

The girls returned from lunch and were gowning up outside the room when I decided to step out and get some lunch myself. As I was leaving, Brenda mentioned in passing that her husband Rich would be there in a few hours. Wait, what? She said he had a job about five hours away and would be moving to Pennsylvania soon. They had clearly been planning this visit and the relocation for a while. In fact, he was already twenty hours into his drive before she informed me of the visit. Rich is a good guy and I would be glad to see him, but the way she went about it really got under my skin. Informing me seemed like an afterthought. I did not blame Rich since I knew this was Brenda showing me that she was going to do what she wanted.

I shouldn't have been, but I was surprised by this move. The way I saw it, she should have checked with me to see if it was okay. Even if she did it in her way by just *telling* me that they were planning it would have been better. It was a courtesy and of course I would not have said no. Suddenly, I was annoyed and getting myself more worked up. Brenda had not spent much time in the room which seemed odd but was starting to make sense as soon as I heard that Rich would be working in the state. I knew that was part of a new plan to move out there. I waited until it was just me and Jessica in the room and asked if Brenda was working on getting her trailer fixed and arranging a move. Jessica confirmed.

My level of aggravation started to rise as I thought about having to deal with this type of thing for months on end. I would have to stress about how she would interact with EVERY single one of our friends visiting. I might show up to find she had a surprise visitor there in Becca's room on any given day. I was done being politically correct with this woman who did not show me (or Rebecca, for that matter) any respect. I did not like the fact that I had to ask so many questions of Jessica but I needed to know what Brenda was scheming.

Brenda had estimated roughly $3,000 to make this happen. If she was collecting donations to cover her costs it would simply be a betrayal. Not only because Rebecca needed it for the transplant fund, but because Rebecca had explicitly made it clear that she did not want Brenda doing this.

A few hours later, my dad and I returned from some errands and Rich and Brenda were sitting in the room. As we walked in and said hello to him he stood up to greet my father and me. I headed toward the far end of the room when something caught my eye. I saw Brenda urgently signaling to Rich that he should stay seated to ensure he kept his seat. "Why?" I thought. Every time the girls had come in, my dad would give up his seat and often head to the waiting room so they would have space. Now she was playing some weird game trying to maintain their position in the room or something.

As we all sat there, Becca received chest PT (a light pounding on her sides with cupped hands). This was nothing new; it had been a routine treatment her entire life. As usual, the monitor would sense the movement as additional heart beats and it would alarm. What was new was that Brenda was freaking out. All of a sudden, the monitor alarmed and she jumped up confused, like she was witnessing a serious medical emergency. It was such a good show that she was actually starting to make Becca anxious. She knew better.

At first I did not know what to make of it but in a few minutes, it dawned on me. She was acting for Rich so he could see how tough this was for her. I saw him looking at her and that it stressed him out. I felt sympathy for him being thrust into this situation.

Normally when Brenda was in the room, she would sit in the most comfortable chair she could find and play on her phone. If the chair was not very comfortable, she would not be there very long. There was not much interaction with Bec outside of casual conversation so I had gotten the sense that she was logging in time. When Bec needed something, Jessica or I would take care of it. We would shave her legs, give her massages, help her eat, basically anything we could do to make her comfortable. If she wanted, we would brush her hair for a half hour but if Brenda pulled hair duty, Bec would get three minutes and a quick bun.

With chest PT done, I walked over to Bec's side where I usually stayed and held her hand. I looked up to see Brenda approach on the other side of the bed and start running her fingers through her hair and looking into her eyes. I was struck by how disingenuous this performance came across while the whole room was looking on.

My cynical side began to emerge. The way I saw it, she felt she had to "sell" this to Rich to justify spending $3,000. She needed her presence to be seen as crucial and helpful. I hated being this way. I wanted to be strong enough to take anything the world could throw at us to ensure a smooth day for Rebecca. Unfortunately, things were coming to a head and I knew our next talk would be even more divisive than the first.

The next morning when they arrived, my dad did not give up his seat. The two of us stayed seated and let the girls stand for a bit. It was not planned but I knew he would not budge after the previous day. I also knew Brenda would not last long. Twenty minutes and she was gone. My dad then got up to give Jessica his seat and we had a nice relaxed morning.

I brought up the trailer discussion, this time with Bec. After I explained the situation, I looked at her and asked do you want your mom living out here? She pondered it for a second and said, "I'm indifferent to it." She had previously been clear that she did not want Brenda there long term and now she was indifferent? I had always been sensitive to Bec's relationship with her mom and tried not to put pressure on her to act in any certain way but this was different. This had been the hardest six months of my life. I sacrificed my job. I had all of the responsibilities for our finances, pets, home, and insurance dealings. I stressed day and night about Bec. My whole life revolved around her and everything I did was for her. Now the person who had made the toughest time in my life even worse, was doing it again and Rebecca was…indifferent?

I could not do it anymore; I could not hold it in. I told her, "I don't know what you want me to do, Bec. You say that you don't care whether she stays or not and you know how she has been with me. I'm let down. You know the way she has acted toward me, talked in anger about me, planned in secret, and that doesn't affect your opinion? Don't say something you don't feel but for somebody whose presence you're saying you don't need, you would just have me deal with her...when you're indifferent?"

If my mom had acted with that much animosity toward Rebecca, I would not have stood for it and my mom had been there for me my whole life. If she was truly "indifferent," wouldn't the rest of these factors give her an opinion? I suppose I expected Becca to defend me, as she acted with Jessica all of those years earlier. Perhaps she did not have the energy to take this fight on but I wasn't looking for that.

I would not allow Brenda to chase me out but realistically, I would probably not be spending as many hours in the room if she was there. It was not a tactic or manipulation, it was reality. I would still come in every day but what kept me in that room for those incredibly long hours was that I was not about to let Rebecca sit there alone. If Brenda was there, I could take more gym time, have a dinner before 9 p.m., or maybe have a morning to sleep in. For that small tradeoff, she could have her mom there and I would suck it up and deal with it. I was willing to roll over or fight the battle myself. I just wanted her direction.

Becca was not okay with me being there even an hour less. She told me that she wanted me there as much as possible. Then she apologized but that was not what I wanted at all and it made me feel worse about having the conversation in the first place. I wanted to feel that she had my back. More than that, I wanted to feel that she was fiercely defensive of me, as I had been of her. I hated this whole conversation. I hated putting Rebecca in this position, especially at this time. In fact, I felt like shit, but everything I said to her was the truth. I did not need her to tell Brenda off, I just needed her support. Tired and disappointed, I asked, "So what do you want?"

"I'm with you." She told me. It was the worst debate that I had ever won.

I decided to talk with Brenda while in the room with Rebecca so there would be no question on her stance. I was ready to go but Brenda was gone for most of the day making her plans in secret. When she finally came back, I waited for the cleaning people to finish, the nurse to administer the meds, and the RT to set up the breathing treatments. I even got up and gave Brenda my seat to ensure she stuck around for a bit. Just as the last person was finishing up, she got up and left again, back to the Family House to "relax." Again I waited.

When she returned a few hours later, the timing was perfect. Sitting by Rebecca's bed, holding her hand, I watched Brenda settle into her normal chair in the corner looking down at her phone. The moment arrived and I just asked her.

"Brenda, are you planning to move out here?"

"No," she said, shocked and indignant.

"So you're not trying to get your trailer fixed up and drive out here?"

"I may bring my trailer out but I'm not moving out."

As I explained that was what I meant, she bobbed and weaved, either slipping the question or dodging the truth. She made it appear that my asking her about her trip was absurd and tried to spin it as though I was telling her she could not see her daughter. I clarified over and over that this was simply about asking us before making plans and I tried to put these boundaries into terms that she could relate to.

"This hospital room is our home, regardless of whether it's here or in Cincinnati. It's the only place I see my wife. We celebrated Easter here. We pay a lot of money to be here. Right now, you are a guest in our home."

"I can't accept that. You've spent more time here but it's not your home." This was not a surprise visit to the ER where people just show up because there is no time to plan. This had been our reality for six months. I shifted the conversation toward how we got here and how informing us of Rich's visit seemed to be an afterthought. I mentioned her secrecy, her rudeness, and her attitude. I simply wanted her to accept that our boundaries would be the same as that of a couple in their home. But time and again she argued, "I can't accept that."

She had asked Jessica to speak with Bec and now wanted her to recount the discussion. Jess was in a tough spot and hesitated. Meanwhile Brenda claimed that Bec would not answer honestly with me there. We were BOTH there and Becca was stronger than that!

I chimed in, "Why don't you just ask Rebecca? Bec, do you want your mom moving out here?" Bec, who had been staring straight ahead, looked over and responded with a clear, "No," to which Brenda started splitting hairs that it was not a move but more of an extended stay. With no hesitation, Becca told her, "I don't want you coming out for an extended stay." For most people, this would halt their plans. Not Brenda. Rebecca pleaded with her mom to just act with respect but Brenda was unfazed.

I reminded her that Rebecca had lost her job and I was losing mine. Bec had needs besides another person in the room and that the $3,000 she needed to raise for her trailer could do more good for Rebecca. She then claimed that her trailer did not need repairs and that everything would be free because it was all "donated." At that point, I proposed she get donations for Bec and she acted like she did not know how to fundraise, though we had seen her do so numerous times for other causes. She then suggested that this was "all about money." Arguing about money was useless and if she lied about not needing repairs, this was going nowhere.

We rehashed January's events and I mentioned how her illness would have risked Rebecca's health had I not stopped her. But in her new version, she was never sick and only had some allergies—weird winter allergies diagnosed three weeks after the fact. What was the point of this discussion if she continued to lie at every turn?

When she repeated that she was coming out to see her daughter I flashed back to that February discussion with Jess. I asked, "Are you sure you're not coming out to look me in the eye and see my body language when you walk through the door?" I stopped talking and just allowed the silence to hang in the air. I needed to let her know that I was aware of her rantings and her "allies." If she was going to rail against me in private, she could not act innocent in front of me. I gave her one last chance to respect our position that this was our home, our bedroom, but she refused.

Finally I told her, "I can't stop you from moving to Pittsburgh…" She nodded, with a little smirk. "But I control who comes into this room because I pay the bills. So if you can't respect that, I will ban you from coming in this room."

I was looking her straight in the eye with an intensity I had never felt before. She stepped back in shock then she turned and looked to Rebecca hoping for an ally. I knew that Bec had my back so I just kept staring at Brenda. In that moment, I did not know Becca's exact response, but I saw the look in Brenda's eyes and watched her body language as reality settled in.

After a moment's pause, she looked back at me, "Okay, I can accept that." She turned to Rebecca, grabbed her other hand and started stroking it.

I did not trust her. She was going to do what she was going to do but she knew, if she did not respect the line I had drawn, she would have to deal with the consequences. I couldn't just *threaten* to ban her from the room in order to get respect, I had to mean it. I meant it.

Before stepping out of the room I told her, "We're good. That was all I was looking for." She was quiet. In the end, I was asking her to respect our boundaries. It took a lot of reflection before I decided to have this conversation. What pushed me over the edge had nothing to do with clearing the air from the past. Much of it seemed like a lifetime ago and though it still frustrated me, I could chalk her actions up to emotion. My motivation was not the present either. I felt disrespected by the lack of communication regarding Rich's visit but we both really liked Rich. But as I considered that, along with her secret trailer plan, it served as a trigger to recognize that things would get worse if I did not put a stop to it.

The true reason for this conversation was the future. Why wouldn't she continue to act this way if she saw nothing wrong with it? I realized that it would become worse as she needed less from me (like housing or transport) so she would probably tell me even less. Justifying whatever she did by saying it was in Rebecca's best interest was an easy out, regardless of whether or not she asked the opinion of her thirty-eight-year-old daughter.

If Rebecca got the transplant, we would have a long road ahead. Was I in for the same treatment every time Rebecca was hospitalized or Brenda got emotional? With a five-year survival rate around 50 percent, many of our better scenarios involved something like this happening again. We needed to lay out the rules and if having the courtesy to ask if it was okay to visit was too much for her pride, then maybe visiting Rebecca was not as important to her as she claimed. I did not think it was cocky to believe that I was a big factor in helping Rebecca maintain her spirits and motivation. I could not do that as well if I was steaming under the surface from being blindsided by Brenda or if I was preoccupied with her attitude. Some may fault me for responding when I did, others would have responded much earlier. There are times to turn your cheek and take the high road and everybody has different levels of what they accept. Once it was apparent that there was no end in sight for her actions, I decided to do something I could not have imagined six months earlier, I drew a line in the sand.

Lesson 33: When you realize that someone's disrespectful actions will continue, address them head-on.

The next day followed with only short appearances from Brenda, totaling less than two hours. I stepped out when she was there so that Becca could get the most from her visit.

Brenda loved her daughter but her pride was stronger. Pride was why she left in January instead of going to St. Louis. Pride was why she never planned a fundraiser and why she stopped texting Becca for two weeks after we told her that it was necessary to go through COTA. Pride was why she wasn't going to ask us to visit our room for the next few months. She would rather to return to Idaho than ASK if it was okay stay. At the beginning of the year I looked forward to impressing her; six months later she had thoroughly disappointed me.

CHAPTER 22

The Offer

After our confrontation, Brenda started leaving earlier and would try to get Jessica to leave around dinnertime so they could eat together. At the same time, I would try to convince Jess to stay because Rebecca really enjoyed it. I felt bad that she was stuck in the middle.

At this point, I was particularly thankful for my father who sat in the waiting room for most of the day, not even asking when we were going to leave. Though the days became increasingly longer, all he would say is, "I'm good, just let me know what you want to do." The next few days, my dad and I would take the early *and* late shifts. It was worth it for the peace of mind I had taken from "The Talk."

This left us there alone the night Becca threw up what mostly looked like blood and blood clots. It was a terrible sight and a reminder that we were living on borrowed time. It had been two weeks and two days on ECMO. It was a hard night to leave but I promised her that I would come in earlier the next morning. I had no idea how much earlier at the time...

At 12:37 a.m. on June 16, my phone rang. It was a Pennsylvania number and in the middle of the night, it could only be extremely good or extremely bad news. I was lying there awake and answered immediately. The voice on the other end of the line told me, "We have an offer for lungs." It was the news I had been waiting to hear for what seemed like an eternity! They still needed to go and evaluate them. They were considered "high risk" which meant they may have participated in high risk activities. In this case it was because the donor had a sexually transmitted infection (nothing that affected the lungs). There was no choice, we were taking them!

She asked if I wanted to come in and sit with Becca or try to get some rest and come in early. The evaluation would be done in the morning so I figured it would be best to get some rest. I lay there tossing and turning for a while, then decided to text her. If she was awake, I would come in, if not I would try (in vain) to sleep. She was awake and excited! I was coming in. I told her that, then immediately got a text from her nurse suggesting I get some rest. I was not coming in.

I started to text everyone about three separate times but then I stopped. There was no point in preventing everyone else from sleeping. It ended up being the best crappy night's sleep I ever had.

They said that "donor time" (when they would look at the lungs) would be at 6:30 a.m. My dad and I were there at 5:30. I walked into her room to see a tube coming out of her nose with tape around it. Was this some sort of prep for the surgery? I remembered that her feeding tube had a leak... The look on the nurse's face suggested something more.

The vomiting last night made them nervous enough to do a bronch, turn off her tube feeds, turn off her heparin, and insert a feeding tube through her nose for an emergency stomach pump if necessary. When he told me that they did not take her off the list and that it should not affect the events of the day, it was reassuring and chilling at the same time. I had not considered that it was a risk. Were we so close to being bumped off the list? It felt like we had used all of our "overtimes." They told us when she got on ECMO she would probably have only two weeks to live. It had been two weeks, two days, and twelve hours.

We waited all morning as anticipation built. The anesthesiologist stopped in to evaluate all of her lines. The clinical research nurse came by to ask if she would participate in a trial. There was an excitement in the air as we eyed everyone near the room as a potential source of information which we hoped was word of final approval.

Rebecca was nowhere nearly as excited as I had expected. At this point, she was very focused on the here and now. She was very uncomfortable from the nasogastric tube and kept asking EVERYONE if they could remove it—the nurse, the RT, the perfusionist, the doctor...it was clear that she did not want that thing in there any longer. It was making her so miserable that she could not really appreciate the events that were unfolding.

It was 9:15 a.m. when I recognized a transplant surgeon, Dr. Jonathan D'Cunha gowning up. He came in and told us that he had reviewed the lungs. I could not read his expression with his mask on but he came out with the verdict quickly. The lungs were no good.

It was a big letdown. I expected that it would take the wind out of my sails but it didn't, completely. I had become pretty good at receiving bad news so I did my best to roll with it. I had gotten myself worked up and was convinced it was going to be a *yes*. Rachel had even called to ask if she should go to work...she had a packed bag and was ready to head out at the drop of a hat.

They had found pneumonia in the lungs and could not use them. Dr. D'Cunha had told us that there could be more dry runs like this because they were looking at all possible lung options including the high risk ones. I looked over at Becca to see how she was doing and she was let down. He asked if we had questions and we did not. Well, Bec had a question, "When can we take this tube out of my nose?"

It was not long before she did get it pulled, after which she seemed happier than that morning when we had hopes for new lungs. As a result, the afternoon was better than I could have expected as we waited around for what seemed as likely as lightning striking a second time.

That night I sat on the couch with my dad, a glass of tequila in hand, watching an action flick, wondering when the next call would come. I had spent the past few hours talking myself up from the day's disappointment. Though it had been a misfire, it helped to drive the point home that it was a real possibility. The call could come at any time and Bec could be in surgery a few hours later.

Not long into the movie I got a call from the hospital. Again, there was a nurse on the line. "I know I called you last night with the same message, but we have another set of lungs we are going to evaluate for Rebecca." This time, there was no caveat about high risk and suddenly, our ordinary tequila turned into celebratory tequila! This time she suggested that I go to bed, get some rest, and come in before 7 a.m. (donor time).

It was time to get worked up all over again. I did not worry about being let down again because I had learned we had to celebrate whatever victories we could because we did not know when the next one would come. The right combination of pre-exhaustion and tequila made sleep much easier that night and we were up and out bright and early again the next morning.

June 17, 2015: Facebook post

We got another call last night about donor lungs. We expected the evaluation to occur at 7AM this morning and I'd be posting an update earlier but the time keeps getting pushed out and is now planned for 8PM. Once the lungs are approved (hopefully), the transplant will take place after the organ transport. No times yet but it could be as early as 6 hours from now!

This time we knew the drill, but instead of an early *no*, we got a lot of delay. Donor time moved from 7 a.m. to 2 p.m. to 7 p.m. to 8 p.m. to 10 p.m. I felt like something was up but nobody we spoke with knew much of anything.

They cancelled all of her chest therapy that day because it was not worth the risk of causing some pulmonary failure. I could see Bec doing everything she could to stay in the fight. She was stuck on this ECMO machine, laying stiff as a board so as to not risk problems with the cannulas. All she could do was listen to the soothing sounds through her sound dampening headphones and stare straight ahead. She had a look in her eye that I had seen before. It was the look of a fighter getting their mind right before a match. It reflected a focus and an intentional calm. Hour after hour that was all she did...look straight ahead while listening to her sounds. I was filled with this sense that it was her last chance at life. We all sat and waited.

Dr. D'Cunha finally came in to speak with us and we waited anxiously to hear what he had to say. The donor lungs had retained some fluid during the day and demonstrated a decreasing blood gas performance. The doctors had been diuresing them to reduce the fluids and the newer gases showed some improvement but not enough. He said that they normally would not send someone out to look at them but because Rebecca was so sick, they would.

So we had a plan. They told us that we might hear back as early as midnight but she could get wheeled out at any time. So we waited there...Bec with her headphones, Dad in the waiting room, Jess and Brenda in the room with us...we just waited.

By this point, it must have been around 9 p.m. The charge nurse came in and told us that they had started removing the lungs. It wasn't a *yes* but it was one step closer. They would still evaluate them upon removal and then again upon arrival at Pittsburgh...so we waited harder.

At about 10:30 p.m., the attending CTICU doctor popped her head through the curtains and gave us a big smile and a thumbs up. We all looked at each other with excitement. Was that a *yes*?!? Say it was a *yes*! Just say something! That doctor must have wasted four entire seconds before telling us that the lungs were good and that Rebecca was going to get her transplant, "Get what you need and hug her good-bye, we need to prep her for surgery!"

I got to her first and hugged her and kissed her, "You're gonna do great!" I could see the excitement and anxiety in her eyes...but we had to go. I grabbed iPads and iPhones, chargers, a pillow, and my Shit Happens bag. Brenda said good-bye and grabbed pillows and blankets from the room...Jessica said good-bye then grabbed whatever was closest to her, mostly medical trash. As we rushed out of there, I hung back to say another good-bye to Becca, shook the hands of a familiar nurse or two, and we were off...Becca to get her new lungs and us to anticipate every update!

I caught up with the girls. "Jess, I grabbed your charger. Why do you have all of that trash?"

"We had to go so I just started grabbing things!"

"Good job."

We found my dad who was now a family lounge expert. We headed to the larger lounge and he immediately identified for us the chair that would not recline, the temperature controls, and the restroom location. As we all got settled in our recliners, I knew there was no way I could go to sleep. I started watching a movie and possibly lasted eight minutes before I was out like a light. I was so exhausted but that was only part of the reason. There was not a question in my mind about the success of this surgery. I knew that it would go well, it had to. In any case, it was out of my hands.

I woke up at 3 a.m. to a tap on the knee. It was the charge

nurse. The first lung was in! Everything was progressing as planned.

I woke up at 6:30 a.m. to another tap, the second lung was in and they were working to get her off of ECMO!

I understood the nature of a lung transplant and that she would receive new lungs that worked, but it was somehow surprising when they told me she would be removed from ECMO. I was in disbelief.

After some texting and posting, we were waiting again for the next update. My phone rang about 9 a.m. and the surgery was done. Dr. D'Cunha wanted to speak with me so I headed off to meet him. Jessica and Brenda were trying to get their things together but I was not patient enough to wait. I took off immediately and went to the wrong room. When I finally realized where I had to go, Jessica and Brenda had caught up. Jessica had employed the same tactic that she used the night before and grabbed everything that was close by. This time, her arms were filled with all of the blankets and pillows we had brought to the lounge. Good job.

As we sat down with the surgeon, I could see that he was pleased with the result, "The surgery went well." He mentioned that she had a lot of scar tissue on the outside of her lungs which made them incredibly difficult to remove. The new lungs however, went in "perfectly." I had rarely heard a doctor use those words.

He spoke a little of the recovery process and risks of complications but the overall message was that the transplant was a success! When he left, Brenda walked over with open arms to hug Jessica and me. The three of us stood in the middle of this waiting room relieved and exhausted. It was an amazing moment.

On June 18, 2015, Rebecca received her double lung transplant. I would forever remain in awe of her amazing caregivers, the state of the art technology, her incredible will, and her fleet of guardian angels that somehow managed to keep her alive. It was truly a miracle.

We were allowed in her room around 10 a.m. and Bec was sleeping. She looked so much more comfortable without the large cannula in her neck and stitched to her leg. We were trying to be quiet but we were all so excited.

She had five chest tubes that were inserted into her chest cavity. These were to collect excess fluid and prevent it from building up and putting pressure on the lungs. The plan was to remove these as the drainage slowed. She also had a breathing tube in her mouth again. This was a special type to oxygenate the new lungs which was why they could not use her trach. Maybe I was just used to seeing this stuff but it looked nowhere near as uncomfortable as it did in January.

Not long after we got there, my dad eased his way back to the waiting room. He needed to make the rounds and tell all of his new friends the good news!

Brenda got up and told us she was going back to Family House for a nap. She was done for the day.

Like so many times that year, it was just Bec's sister and me in there, watching her sleep. Jessica suggested I go to the gym. I thought it was a great idea and even told her I would take her up on it, but as the hours passed, I could not bring myself to leave. I just sat there in amazement and disbelief of what had just happened. I knew the road to recovery would be long, but we had already been through that process once, and the first time our best hope was to live long enough in hopes to get transplanted...and the odds were against us. This time, our goal was a full recovery and the odds were looking pretty good. There was this huge weight lifted from my shoulders. My other concerns could wait because the biggest worry was resolved...she had her new lungs!

She would wake up for short periods here and there. Her main problem was that she was not comfortable. She did not complain much of pain, which seemed unusual to me. However, seeing as this was the first transplant I had witnessed, I may not have been a subject matter expert. When she finally did start complaining of pain, it was in the early evening. She told us of this pain she was feeling *here*. She pointed at her chest.

I asked her if her chest hurt and she nodded *yes* with a sad expression on her face. Jessica lightly placed her hand on her chest and said, "It hurts because you have these new beautiful lungs in there. The pain you're feeling is from the transplant." Rebecca's eyes were closed but we could see tears start to pool in the corners.

"Did you know that you've got beautiful new lungs...that you got the transplant?!" Jessica asked.

Rebecca shook her head *no*.

"Are those tears of joy?"

Rebecca nodded her head *yes*. You could see the corners of her mouth pulling back as they did when she would cry. It was an unbelievable moment.

Jessica and I looked at each other and back at Bec. We were on either side of the bed and were both holding a hand. It felt amazing to be a part of this moment...there was no other place in the world I would have rather been!

The next couple of days were a blast. She had received a lot of sedation so we expected we would be in for a treat with all of her questions and requests. She did not let us down. It was hard to read her lips while she was intubated and her handwriting was still horrible. Not to mention that she had trouble forming the thoughts in her head to begin with.

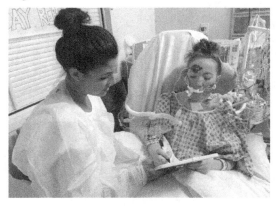

On her dry erase board, she asked us, "What is the humidity?" Then she underlined "humidity." Then she added, "In the room?" She had this level of urgency about her with which we were quite familiar. I stepped up and told her that the humidity was 60 percent. That satisfied her briefly, and then she thought for a second and asked, "How do you know that, where is the gauge?"

"You got me, Bec, I don't know what the humidity is."

She gave me the side eye, thought for a second, and then modified her message wiping off *humidity* and replacing it with *blood pressure*. I read it off to her, "What is the blood pressure in the room?"

She shook her head *yes* and I read it to her. That seemed to satisfy her. She essentially wanted to know that her numbers were good but was just having a tough time determining which numbers to ask about.

A short time later, the nurse asked her if she wanted to get in a chair. Very seriously she mouthed, "What's my blood pressure?" We told her and confirmed it was good then she said, "Okay, I'll get in the chair."

"Don't worry, Bec, they wouldn't move you if your numbers weren't good enough," I told her. Jess and I looked at each other with a smile.

Sitting in the chair she told Jessica, "Put your hands under my feet, under my skin." She wanted us to support her feet so she could push herself up in the chair. Sedation Becca just had a way with words...this quote was good enough to be another "Hey Deere, ASAP!?????"

June 19, 2015: Facebook post

In January, during the first few days Rebecca was in the ICU, my thoughtful sister Rachel sent me a care package. There were quite a few helpful items for both of us contained in this "Shit Happens" colon cleanse bag.

The bag seemed oddly appropriate and I started taking it to and from the hospital every day. I used it for just about everything at one point or another…legal papers, food, gym clothes, a cooler, bills, my iPad, travel mugs…everything. I learned a key lesson that coffee and legal papers are not a good combination in a bag like this. As time passed, it inspired me to dress better to ensure that I wouldn't look like a homeless person carrying it around.

Today, we are so thankful to have the transplant behind us…and though we still have a long road to recovery ahead, it's time for me to retire the "Shit Happens" bag. Goodbye old friend, it looks like some of the bad shit has stopped happening ;)

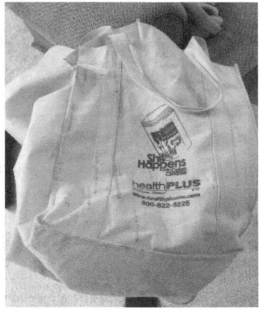

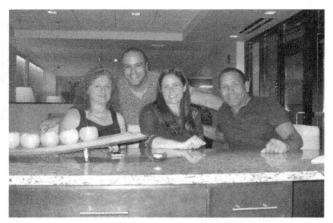

The next days seemed to race by. With a few more visitors, we would spend our days in the hospital and our nights celebrating.

From Left to right: Louise, Ray, Rachel, Ray (Sr.)

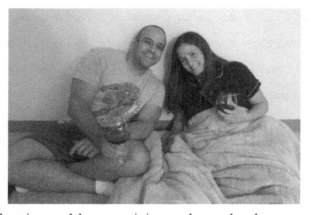

Rachel and I even got to drink classy red wine on the floor!

The only issue that seemed to be of concern was Becca's kidney function. She was not making enough urine and her creatinine and urea levels were out of range. They said that kidney failure was a risk going into the surgery, primarily because of the rejection meds and the fact that her kidneys were not that great to begin with. However, when the renal doctors came in, they suggested that this was likely due to a drop in blood pressure that occurred during the surgery. This could cause acute injury to the kidneys.

This was the first time I heard them mention dialysis. It was concerning and I could imagine us at home, not able to leave the house for long periods because she needed to return for dialysis. I could imagine a lot, particularly because I knew nothing about dialysis. Regardless, I just hoped that she would not require it. They explained that if she did require it, her kidneys could potentially recover. Also, a typical treatment plan was three to four hours, three times per week. As I rationalized it to myself, this was nothing compared to what she had been through, particularly ECMO. They could provide a more comfortable catheter if it became long term and she could arrange to come into the hospital for her treatments. So, if that was the worst case scenario, it was nothing compared with what we had been facing.

The next test confirmed that she required it. One doctor explained that her kidneys needed some time to "wake up" from the surgery. We were also concerned that the anti-rejection medication was tough on the kidneys and often caused some issues on their own. There were no tough decisions to make. They would just treat her and wait to see how her body responded.

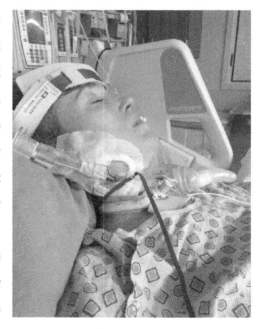

They placed the catheter in the right side of her neck and brought in two large machines. One was to process the water required and the other did the work of pumping and processing her blood. The technician allowed me to stay in the room and answered all of my questions on how it worked. An added benefit was that it typically made people sleepy and she was getting it at night. Conveniently, it might actually result in a good night's sleep for a change.

Instead of following the original plan for three consecutive days of dialysis followed by every other day, they were able to skip the second day. This was a good sign. We saw her urinating more and some slight improvements showed in her numbers. After her second treatment, they postponed the third one twice, and then cancelled it altogether. So after only two treatments, her kidneys had recovered and she was off of dialysis.

CHAPTER 23

The Healing Factor

It was exciting to see all of the tubes and lines start to come out. This was an exciting time as she lost her neck IVs, dialysis catheter, and some of her chest tubes, all while becoming more alert and gaining strength. During the days she was placed on a trach mask, a mask that fit over her tracheostomy site delivering humidified oxygen. Nothing was connected or providing any pressure support, it was just this tube blowing oxygen near her trach while she did the work of breathing.

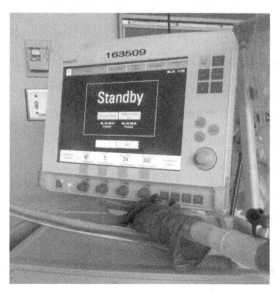

She had been on a ventilator for 171 days then suddenly, a day after transplant, she was off it. Even if only for a few hours at a time, it was remarkable. All of the worries of the tube popping off and not catching it in time vanished.

The team increased her time on the trach mask daily until she was on it for the full day.

Once they determined she was ready, they switched her to BiPAP at night which is a machine typically used for sleep apnea. So within a week of the surgery, she was completely off the ventilator. The transplant team had spent a lot of time telling us about the long road to recovery, but after what we had just been through, it was progressing rapidly by comparison.

Her biggest complaint was that she could not eat anything. I remember coming in one morning to find her in tears as she told me that it would be three weeks before she could eat. She told me that she was STARVING! All I could do was remind her that she was getting her nutrition from the tube feeds and try to comfort her. They were particularly cautious in this hospital about eating on a trach and they definitely did not want her to aspirate into these new lungs.

Aside from the risk of choking and infection, aspiration could promote rejection which was the biggest fear we had going into the transplant. Rejection occurs when the body attacks the transplanted organ as a reaction to a foreign object. To avoid this, they had her on several anti-rejection meds that basically compromised her immune system to prevent it from damaging her lungs. This was a balancing act because she still kind of needed an immune system...

Every morning before her snoozer, they would take a trough, which was a blood draw timed when blood levels of her main anti-rejection med (tacrolimus) were at a minimum. They tried to maintain levels within an optimal range. Depending on her daily levels, they would increase or decrease her dosage. She also took medication to prevent fungal and bacterial growth. We thought she was on a lot of medications previously, but the post-transplant list was several pages long.

Either all or some combination of her handful of morning pills would make her nauseous. Not surprisingly, that did not support the goal of switching to food by mouth. She had sufficient calories and nutrition but that was not enough. She felt hungry and craved her favorite foods...and coffee.

Though I felt for her, I did not feel *bad* for her which was a nice, subtle change. There was so much positive progress during these days that even though it was fine to recognize the challenges, we could not let it rule our moods. Of course that was easy for me to say after I had my eggs and steel cut oats that morning.

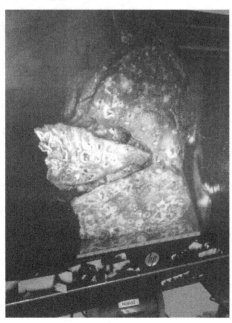

It was in her room in the MICU where we finally saw pictures of her old lungs. We got to see these worn out, battered organs that had squeaked by and lasted her *barely* long enough, but long enough. They showed us on the monitor and it was astonishing. These beat up, scarred and burned up looking things somehow managed to keep her alive. It was a miracle. I could tell that Rebecca was thinking the same thing because when I turned back to look at her, her expression said it all…

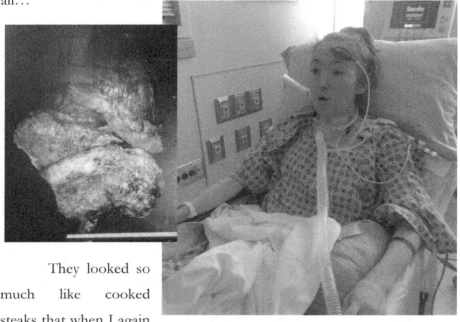

They looked so much like cooked steaks that when I again showed her the pictures of them, she commented on how they looked good. Maybe it was her hunger talking, but she changed her tune when I clarified that they were her lung photos. She had come a long way!

We soon got some exciting news as she achieved a new milestone. They decided to transfer her to the ninth floor…the transplant recovery floor. For the first time in almost two months she was out of the ICU! The nurse told us that it would be any minute so I packed up and brought our gear upstairs to organize it in our new digs. I headed up with toiletries, socks, hair products, and the big balloon I got her with a frog on it that said, "HOPE TO SEE YOU HOPPING AROUND SOON!"

After about forty-five minutes of sitting in the room with a frog balloon, I felt like a kid at his eighth birthday party slowly coming to the realization that his friends were not coming. Well, I suppose I knew they were coming but I was clearly more excited about this move than anyone else so I was not going to continue to sit there alone. Though it happened on hospital time, it eventually happened and we transferred to a room with an actual door. It signified moving to a situation where a get well soon card would actually feel applicable. It was the first time this year that rest and PT would move us toward actual recovery.

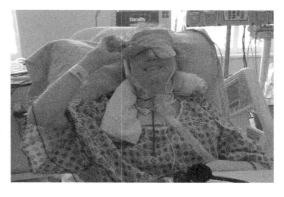

Soon my mom and niece, Ashley, came out to visit. They got to see her walk and she looked great. I did not like the fact that her sats were floating around 93 percent that day because they had been pinned at 100 percent since the transplant. The doctors explained that there would be ups and downs so I guess we would just wait for them to come back up.

That night we went home and were sitting down to a movie when my phone rang. I recognized that it was a hospital number and I knew they could not be calling with good news. I answered the phone to have my fears confirmed. Rebecca had desatted badly, down into the 50s, and her CO_2 level rose significantly as well. She was rushed back to the CTICU and hooked back up to a ventilator. They could not tell me anything for certain, but one of the potential causes was rejection.

After all of the highs from the past week and a half, this was like getting the wind knocked out of me. When we arrived the next morning, she was on the ventilator. I needed to remind myself that two steps forward and one step back had brought us this far. There was a bronch scheduled for that day which we hoped would shed some light on what had happened.

Not long after they wheeled her out, I received a call from the nurse. They were looking for approval from me for the procedure. This was a bit odd because Bec was awake when she left but I gave the approval and did not give it a second thought...until the nurse came back and tried to relax me. "The only reason we needed it was because Becca seemed disoriented. We think her CO_2 level rose during the transport."

This certainly did not relax me! So in the fifteen minutes it took to bring her there, her CO_2 level went high enough to disorient her? Now I was really starting to get concerned. This all felt like uncharted territory. We hoped for an answer when she returned from the bronch but got none. The nurse was told that the bronch "went well" which could mean many things. I took it to mean that there were no problems during the procedure. It would be days before any real results came so it was time again to wait harder.

When the doctor came by to explain, he used a term to describe some tissue that I had not heard yet. He was talking quickly but it stood out because it started with *necro* which I knew meant dead. So some kind of dead tissue was found in her new lungs but we still did not know if that was a result of rejection or something else. As we sat in the room absorbing all of this, my mom asked me if I knew how to get to the ER.

"What's going on?" I asked, suspecting it was related to migraines and high blood pressure issues she had experienced in the past.

"I just want to get checked out. I have a pain in my neck and I'm getting these heart palpitations since I got here. They're not going away."

I took her there and luckily, Ashley was there to stay with her while I returned to Becca's room hoping another doctor would arrive to give me more news. Within a few hours, Bec was down for the night and I returned to the ER for the latest with my mom. There were several issues: her potassium was low, she had been getting neck pain, and had elevated blood pressure along with these palpitations. They recommended that she stay for observation. She protested but ultimately agreed. Now we had two people in the hospital. At least we just had one place to go to visit them.

The next day we floated between upstairs and down while we waited for news on my mother and my wife. Finally we got some movement as they released my mom with a monitor to record her vitals for forty-eight hours. I knew it was the stress of making the drive that affected her as travel often did. I was just glad to have one issue resolved!

Meanwhile, Rebecca got to walk and was placed back on a trach mask for short intervals. We did not have any additional instances of dropping sats or elevated CO_2 so we anxiously awaited the explanation. All seemed to be good with her over the next couple of days but I did not have that warm and fuzzy feeling. With no root cause, we did not know if this issue could crop up out of the blue again. Was this tied to some larger issue that would get worse? My fear was that it was the start of rejection.

Rejection came in two forms: acute and chronic. Immediately after the transplant, we were concerned with acute. Chronic manifested over time. This is one of the reasons why the first year is so critical for lung transplant patients. Another day went by and finally, the doctor came by with the biopsy results. There was no rejection. Thank God. There was no rejection.

So…what happened? What could cause her lungs to stop working if there was no rejection? Injury. We were told that some kind of lung injury may have been the cause. It could have happened before the transplant when they were outside the body and symptoms were just manifesting. Ultimately, we didn't know.

That was the frustrating thing about much of what had gone on this year. There was not a test for everything so they eliminated what they could, using the tests at their disposal. After that, we could only use logic to deduce the rest. After watching *House* for several seasons, I knew this was the best answer we were going to get.

It was a good answer. It explained what happened and also suggested it was unlikely to reoccur. They would just watch her closely, performing bronchs more frequently over the next couple of weeks. Another day and she would go back to the ninth floor…back to recovery.

Up until this point, she was not allowed to drink water, only allowed to swish and then suck it out with a tube called a yonker. She did not comply with this for very long and soon would just swallow the water. Shortly after that she started eating "illegal" ice. It was there to keep her sterile water cold but she was a rebel. She would grab pieces and crunch away to her heart's content.

One day, the aide caught her and instead of admitting guilt, she put on her most innocent expression and mouthed, "I didn't know that, nobody told me!" She had these sad little wrinkles on her forehead that not only expressed her innocence, but her aversion to doing anything outside the rules...even unknowingly. I would have believed her if I did not already know that she was lying through her teeth. Good form, Rebecca, good form!

Rachel and her family came out to visit next. Rebecca was back on her trach mask and her BiPAP was cut to four hours a night. Aside from moving forward medically, she seemed to be more herself. It was great to see her chat with Rachel and Gabrielle and laugh when Justin and Jeremy goofed around with Michael. It was night and day compared to Easter, and instead of the bittersweet mood of that holiday, this visit had more energy. Visits at this point were no longer a potential last good-bye. They had shifted to being more reminiscent. Though I had lost track of whom I had told what stories to, I was pretty certain that the kids and Michael had not heard most of them so I was not repeating them for a change.

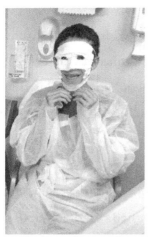 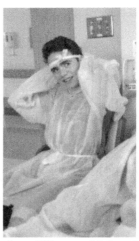

We talked about the good times we would have when Becca was discharged. For her it was a nice distraction from being uncomfortable or stuck in her room. She still nodded off now and again but she really enjoyed our family time together. We would head home for lunch, and then back to the hospital still trying not to leave Becca for long periods. This was tough because our large group moved slowly and could easily get distracted by conversation. We ate some good steaks, drank some nice wine, enjoyed great conversation, and looked forward to each day.

When the time finally came for them to say good-bye I suggested that Bec stand up to hug everyone. It seemed simple but for months, everybody had only hugged her in her chair or her bed. Not only did she stand up but she started dancing. As everyone rotated through for their good-byes, she danced between each and every one. She was strong. Seeing her so happy and being goofy was uplifting for everyone.

Back at the apartment, that was all we could talk about. It was a moment etched in all of our memories, mine in particular because it had been so long since I had seen her happy enough to celebrate and strong enough to dance.

My new daily routine involved a little less rushing and a lot less dread. Unfortunately, my relaxed mornings were not appreciated when Rebecca was uncomfortable. One morning, she texted me and asked when I would arrive. I was right down the hallway but I typed that I might be a while. Then less than a minute later, I stopped in to surprise her.

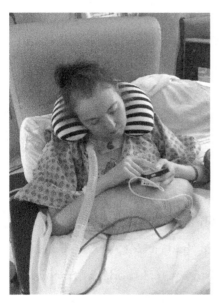

This woman could fall asleep on a dime. She had texted me then immediately passed out! Her phone did not even have enough time to shut off before she did. I could see why there was such urgency...her pillows were a mess and comfort is the first priority when you are stuck in a chair all day long.

Progress continued as they changed her trach for one that was a smaller size. This was significant because it could be fitted with a speaking valve allowing her to talk. The next step after this was the swallow test...and EATING! This was sure to lift her spirits.

After the first day with the new trach, her voice had only returned partially. A quick scope identified that her vocal chords had reduced in size and one side no longer moved. It sounded concerning as they explained this but they had a potential fix. They would inject her vocal chords with a substance to essentially inflate them. It was a temporary fix that was expected to last about three months but it could give them enough time to recover the rest of the way on their own.

She would not be able to talk for two days (including mouthing words) and I kept joking with her that this would be a nice break for me. In reality, it created a situation with no winners. She would start to talk, I would remind her not talk, and then she would get annoyed at me. The other down side was that her swallow test would get pushed out a few more days. It had now been a month since the transplant and she was desperate to eat real food.

By July 21st, they were ready to remove her trach. They were so confident that she would not be back on a ventilator in the near future that it could come out. It was amazing and scary at the same time because it was our safety net. By this point however, it was capped and she was breathing through her nose with only the help of some supplemental oxygen, so the time was right.

As the next weeks passed, we had a lot of incremental improvements. She was finally approved to eat real food, her trach was removed, and she was taken off BiPAP requiring only supplemental oxygen. As the need for oxygen waned, we focused on walking two, then three, then four times a day.

I wrote her workouts up on the board in her room so that Bec could see her accomplishments. My other motivation was to give her a tool to quickly communicate her activity level to any new caregiver. Often someone unfamiliar with her work ethic would tell her to walk more which was a huge pet peeve for her. She needed to be recognized for the work she did.

Nothing frustrated her more than somebody telling her that she was not doing enough when she was exceeding her targets. We would not only walk with pulmonary rehab and physical therapy, we would walk on our own to ensure we hit the target. It

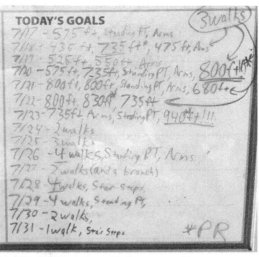

was a bit cumbersome with the IV pole, drainage collectors, and oxygen but I developed a pretty slick system and we made it happen.

It was five weeks post-transplant and she still had drainage tubes that were putting out way too much fluid. They had been able to remove four chest tubes and two blakes (smaller tubes) but one chest tube remained...and remained...and remained. We definitely did not want to pull it too soon because the body would continue to produce fluid with nowhere for it to go. We did not want that fluid pressing on the lungs preventing them from fully expanding. The question remained: why is she producing so much?

They said this sometimes occurred with younger patients and CF patients, so that made me feel a little better. They also test the fluid for infection and to see if the surgeon(s) may have nicked a gland during the procedure but it all looked good. I supposed that boiled down to the answer: It doesn't matter.

I constantly reminded her of what things would be like when

we got to the apartment and I knew she was looking forward to it.

The days did get long sometimes and it was hard for other people to understand that recovery was challenging even if things seemed good. I would post mostly the positive things on Facebook but for some reason I occasionally found myself irritated when some comments suggested that the problems were all resolved. I knew they were feeling relieved for us and this came from good intentions. However, I also knew we had many more challenges to face. I found myself reading into the comments that I had 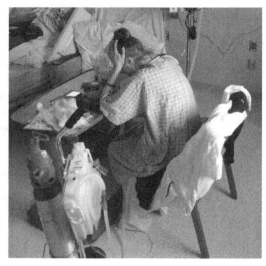 nothing to complain about because all of my prayers were answered.

It is not that I like to complain, on the contrary, I prided myself on the fact that I kept it to a minimum, but I wanted to reserve the right to do so. Rebecca had received a lifesaving transplant but the five-year survival rate was only about 50 percent. I treasured every day I had with Bec but I had not taken a day for myself since this insanity had started and there was no such thing as a weekend for me. We had enough money in the bank for the time being but we were both unemployed and whittling our savings away. I could return to work but it meant leaving her at home and I risked losing that job if Bec suddenly required a few weeks back at UPMC.

Work was a recurring worry for me. I did not know when it would be safe to start looking for a job. If I found a job, I would need one that required less of my time and less travel, which would likely result in less pay. I could not work the twelve-hour days and partial weekends while I worried about Rebecca at home. I could very likely be pulled away from work at a moment's notice by another health crisis and lose my job again.

I had spent years building a career and this would be a major setback. We always knew that Rebecca would stop working at some point but I never anticipated the problems her CF could pose to my career...and therefore to our livelihood. We had just purchased a beautiful home that we planned to stay in for many years and now I wondered if we would be forced to sell it. I wanted to be able to utilize this time to be together because I did not know how much time we had.

The closer we came to discharge, the more I thought about work. I knew it would be a while before I could do anything about that because we would need to remain in the Pittsburgh area until the doctors felt she was healthy enough to safely move home. Normally this would require a couple of months but we should not be surprised if it took more time since she was so sick and weak prior to transplant.

With discharge pending, I decided to take one last trip home. I asked Rebecca if there was anything in particular that she wanted me to bring from home. She told me that I needed more shirts.

Despite my boring wardrobe, I was riding pretty high on my cloud. Not even the city bus that sideswiped our car could bring me down. I was even looking forward to my quick stop home in order to check on the house and get some of Rebecca's things. It had been a month and a half since I had been home. I was up and out bright and early with a tight yet achievable schedule.

I arrived home to a beeping. The company that built our house decided that there needed to be eighteen different smoke and carbon monoxide detectors in our upstairs foyer so it took me way too many tries to find the right one. As I finally nailed that down, I heard running water. I went into the guest bathroom to find that a basket with shampoo and conditioner that was suctioned to the shower wall had come loose, fallen, hit the faucet on the way down and turned on the water. I was not sure how long it had been on, but mold had started to grow on part of the tub so it was clearly a while.

When I got downstairs, I decided to get a quick snack and maybe watch some TV before I got down to business with all of the errands. I hit the power button and the TV did not turn on. After a few tries it was clear that the power outage my neighbors had posted about was accompanied by a surge that was stronger than my surge protector and definitely stronger than my TV since it was fried. That would probably cost more than my pending water bill.

After finding a delicious can of beans, I decided to move to the basement and watch TV there. I hit the power button and the TV turned on, but there was no signal. After a long wait with DirectTV service, I discovered that a GFI outlet must have been tripped. It would not have been too bad but the only reason I had maintained service was because I thought I was recording my favorite shows.

Since watching TV was a bust, I figured I would transfer the contents from the downstairs fridge so I could unplug it and save some electricity. Evidently, our tripped GFI turned it off for us. I opened the freezer to a shit-ton of mold and nastiness. A year earlier, Rebecca had purchased a hundred dollars' worth of high-calorie chocolate ice creams. It was about a month before she stopped liking chocolate ice cream. Fortunately for her, she would never have to eat them.

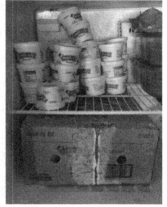

After a nauseating refrigerator cleaning, it only took two quick hours to buff out the car damage from the bus and I could start working on my actual agenda. It was a long day.

Thankfully, nothing in that barrage of crappiness was insurmountable. Everything could be repaired, cleaned, or replaced. Rebecca was off the ventilator, almost out of the hospital, and we were moving toward better days. One thing that this year had provided was perspective. It did not make the events of the day any better but it did help me let them go more quickly. It held a reminder of what I had learned earlier that year...finding a way to appreciate each day meant that I could be annoyed, but I had to be thankful that we were both blessed with health and a promise of more days.

As August approached, so did the first big fundraiser back in Connecticut. I had been looking forward to attending but after months of being in the hospital and under twenty-four-hour care, it suddenly seemed like Rebecca would be discharged that weekend. If that happened, we would be getting her settled into our apartment in Pittsburgh at that time and I would need to stay with her from then on.

Fortunately, Scott was planning to come out for another visit so I had an opportunity to coordinate times. I asked him to come out during the first week in August and stay through the following weekend. I still felt a lot of anxiety to leave her alone but she had been doing so well for so long. She was getting stronger and could move around well. I had also bought several medical aids to help her around the house. She would have a commode, a shower chair, and a rolling walker among other things. The apartment building had ramps and elevators while our unit was all set up with the essentials. There was no reason to worry as long as she had someone with her but it was hard not to.

Scott arrived shortly before she was discharged and Rebecca was so happy to see him. He walked in and they fell into a warm embrace. I quickly felt much better about my trip knowing that she was in good hands.

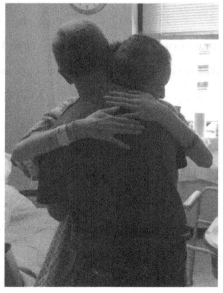

After 218 days in the hospital, Rebecca was coming home. We had been moving toward this day but it was still hard to believe once it happened. On August 5th, she was finally discharged.

We set her up in the apartment and met her new home nurse

Allison that night. With all of her pills, treatments, and home IVs it was nice to have a couple of days to develop a routine before I left. It was really more for my peace of mind than for Scott and Bec because they were both perfectly capable of handling this without me.

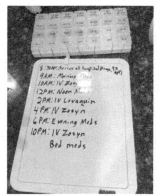

After waiting so long for her to come home, it was really hard to leave. At the same time however, I was excited about the event. Like the overprotective mom I had become, I left them with a filled pill case and detailed instructions on her dry erase board.

The fundraiser was fantastic. Rachel had a small group helping her organize and collect raffle items and they were hugely successful. It was nice getting help from old friends like my buddy Brian and Rachel's friends Jackie and Paul, but what surprised me was all of the help she got from those with whom I had not been as close.

Two ladies, Sara and Karen, who I had not known very well back in high school, helped gather raffle items from local businesses and from high school alumni near and far. One of them commented that it was one of the things she liked about being from a small town: we could all be there to support one another. This was amazing to me. People I had not seen in years arrived from all over Massachusetts, Connecticut, and New York. I could not help but feel incredibly supported and exceptionally blessed surrounded by friends and family.

On this night, my job was to party and talk to everyone—my type of responsibility! Things could not have gone better as we had a strong showing, fantastic prizes, and a great result. In addition to this event, we had sold almost one hundred T-shirts, Meg had run a Jamberry party,

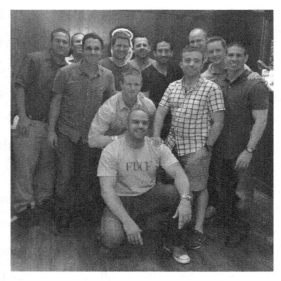

our friend Christy planned an Ava Anderson Fundraiser, Cheryl from my high school did a race, and another friend Vilma released a video for "Fight Song" dedicated to Rebecca with clips showing her journey. Even the flat tire on my ride home was not enough to rain on this parade.

Lesson 34: Never underestimate the boost you can get from the support of others.

Returning home, it seemed like Rebecca was even stronger. Instead of four planned walks, she would walk in the neighborhood. The commode would not come to her, she had to get up and walk to the bathroom multiple times a day. She got a ton of exercise from just puttering around in the kitchen. She quickly became much stronger than I had expected.

CHAPTER 24

FREEDOM

On longer walks, she was using her new rolling walker called a rollator. It had a hand brake, a seat if she got tired, and a basket that was probably too small to hold whatever she was going to buy. I tried to name it Big Red like my dad's old muscle car but the name didn't stick. It was known simply as The Rollator (emphasis on the ROLL).

I had previously scouted other rollator users in the neighborhood and was confident that between her training and her newer model, she could easily take any of them. Knowing that competition would be good for her, I told her, "If you find yourself at a crosswalk and the person next to you has a rollator, do not be afraid to look over and lock eyes. Nobody here has the 'spark'…you can rule these streets." Despite her clear advantage, she had little interest in racing. Perhaps the other rollators steered clear or there were few opportunities—it was hard to say.

Regardless, we took to the streets daily for at least one walk to any of the local coffee shops. This was what we had looked forward to during all of those days in the hospital but her pain and lack of energy often made it feel like less of a treat. She was quiet most of the time and her motivation to talk was if she needed something rather than to share any thoughts. We spoke about where we would go for dinner or what we would do that day. I did not push the subject of discussing the past because I figured she would talk when she was ready.

I tried to keep her focused on these little trips and what was ahead but this remained challenging. We had only been discharged for slightly over a week yet she had a rush of negative feelings and anxiety when she thought about her time in the hospital. This apprehension resurfaced whenever she thought about going in to the hospital, even for a brief appointment. We thought she might have some level of post-traumatic stress disorder. As weeks passed, she would remain in this quieter mood. While she seemed to be stuck in a funk, I was mostly just happy that she was alive, not on a ventilator, and maintaining a positive prognosis. We were certainly not in the same place.

I am not sure if it was depression, but she was not very happy. The reality of her new lungs had not fully sunk in even though it had been almost two months since the transplant. It was becoming clearer to me that she was not focused on her improvements and that she might not come out of this depression any time soon. My goal had become putting a smile on her face. When I succeeded, it did not last long but it was worth it.

The best thing I could throw at her (figuratively) was good food. One night I planned to grill some bacon wrapped fillets along with asparagus. As she sat on the patio chair to wait for dinner, it was apparent that this was not about to make a dent in her mood. I kept trying to start conversations to get her talking but she did not have much to say about anything. I considered that my efforts to get her talking were more annoying than helpful. I was not trying to get her to talk about anything tough...I just wanted her to talk about something or get interested in anything.

I could only keep the conversation going for so long in the face of her complete apathy. I decided I was not going to make idle chit chat anymore. After weeks of this, I was frustrated and if she did not want to talk, I would not bother her. As I started to grill, I thought that maybe I would just shut up for a bit. If she wanted to talk she would. I had been expecting the talkative, excitable Becca to emerge eventually. What I found was the introverted, contemplative, woman from late 2014...the woman who had been busy with work, stressed about the slow process of unpacking our new home, and too exhausted to do much else. I had assumed that the removal of work stress, a clean new apartment, and healthy new lungs would help but they did not.

After all that I had learned from this experience, I almost expected her to have the same takeaways. In retrospect, that would not have made sense. We had been on two different journeys that changed us both. We may have sat in the same hospital room, but my experience was one of coping, waiting, supporting, strategizing...while Rebecca's was simply one of survival.

I felt a desire to discuss with her what I had learned but I sensed that it would not matter until she figured some things out on her own. I did not want to talk seriously before she was ready so I would often wait for her to initiate more serious discussions unless I was giving her a pep talk.

Back in the apartment after our quiet dinner, Bec was preoccupied with her phone while I sat there overthinking our situation. She finally broke the silence but it was to complain about leg pain, stomach pain, tiredness, and nausea. Her feet hurt and she asked me to rub them. As I sat there rubbing her feet, I realized something: she was not dealing with the past or focused on some major trepidation about the future. She was focused on the here and now, and she was uncomfortable. Focusing on the here and now got her through her toughest moments so who was I to say she should change? How could I allow myself to be annoyed by this?

After her foot rub, I gave her a long hug while we stood there in the kitchen. She looked mentally and physically exhausted. I had been patient with her physical recovery. I needed to be more patient with her mental recovery even though I had no idea how long it would take or how I could help. We still had a long way to go. As we started to prep for bed, Bec complained again about being tired then told me that I turned out the wrong light first. I asked her if she was having a bad night and she didn't know. She was having a bad night. As hard as it was, I could not take this personally. I could support her as best I could but I also had to give her space.

Lesson 35: Mental recovery, like physical recovery, takes time and requires a surprising amount of patience.

She was also not pleased with how she looked. One of her post-transplant medications was prednisone. In addition to driving higher blood sugar levels, it also made her retain fluid. As with many people on this medication, it rounded out her cheeks. Clinically this is referred to as moon-face but it really wasn't that bad. The dose would be decreased over time and her chipmunk cheeks would go back to normal but I was anxious for her to be happy with her appearance again…or at least not unhappy.

Mornings were rough as well. She was never a morning person but they were particularly hard after getting discharged. She required a lot of sleep and was awake for only eight to nine hours a day. The morning would come with aches and pain along with nausea. She would come out of the room around 1 p.m. and start the day saying that she felt so lazy for sleeping so long. All I could tell her was that her body must need all of that sleep. She would wander out of the room with her wild sleep hair and her little matching sweat suit. I tried not to smile too much at Morning Becca because it would be received with a glare, but she was a sight. Every morning it looked like she woke from a six-week coma.

She would head straight for the couch and lay back down. She was always in pain but sometimes her head would hurt more than her stomach or her back would hurt less than her chest. I would try to get her to tell me the source of her pain because the next step was to get her to eat some food or do her nebulized treatments. I told her she had to choose one or the other and eventually she would select one depending on what bothered her least that morning. This decision would affect much of the rest of the day as well. If she did her treatments, she would wait even longer to eat, risking more nausea. If she ate first, a stomach ache could delay the nebs resulting in another nap and a shifted schedule. I learned that neither path was better than the other so all I could do was make sure she chose something.

September 30, 2015: Blog Post

Dancing and Vomiting—A story about your dreams coming true…
then throwing up a bit.

Double lung transplant recipients like my wife, have to deal with a lot of challenges but false advertising should not be one of them. Pictured here, is a medication that she was prescribed by her doctor to stop nausea that she unfortunately experiences almost every day. It is called Ondansetron (pronounced "On-DANCE-a-tron"). There is a slight possibility that it is not pronounced this way but I do not care.

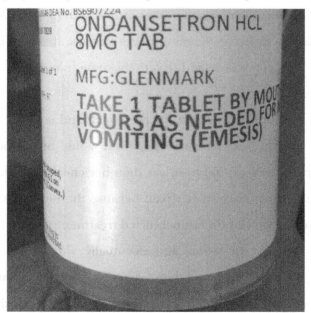

While she is On 'DANCE-a-tron', an insinuated side effect would be

---

that she could become elated and feel strong urges to dance more frequently. I am sorry to tell you, that is not the case and has never been the case with this mislabeled drug!

Typically every morning shortly after Rebecca wakes up, she experiences pain and nausea. We are three months out from her double lung transplant and she understandably still has a fair amount of pain which has fortunately been diminishing slowly week over week. Some of her stomach issues have resolved but it is unpredictable if and when a meal will upset her.

She has cystic fibrosis which can increase digestion issues and stomach pain. This has become worse over the years but we have worked to figure out the cause. Going gluten free seems to have helped but gastrointestinal issues can pop up at any time. We manage space between meals, the types and quantity of foods, and have even experimented with OTC and natural remedies.

A drug name so incredible suggests that it could overcome any propensity that her digestive tract has for acting up, and make her feel so good that she wants to dance. I will say that being on Dance-a-tron helps take the edge off these issues when they come up, though it does not resolve them immediately or completely. I would not expect any drug to be perfect in this respect and it does seem to help if she can take it quickly enough.

However, it is frustrating to see her laying on the couch, in pain and discomfort waiting for the nausea to pass when all logic points to the fact that she should be dancing. Don't get me wrong, we have danced since the surgery and she has had some good mornings. There is nothing better than stringing together a few solid hours and her comfort level has been MUCH better when compared to earlier this year. But…I am still waiting for that key moment when Becca is dancing through most of the day.

Being on dance-a-tron is not all it's cracked up to be. We will continue to try to figure out how to resolve the root cause of the nausea. Though that will ultimately mean no longer being on dance-a-tron, it might lead to more actual dancing.

I planned to write a stern letter to the manufacturer but now that I've spent my free time writing this, it'll have to wait. In either case, I'll continue posting updates to the Facebook page "The Rebecca Martello Poole Lung Transplant Journey" while using this forum for longer posts.

There were so many ways that I wanted to see Rebecca dancing again but I continued to wait, hoping her pain would subside and give her enough of a mental boost to spring back. I knew that once she felt better, some of these other issues would begin to fade.

Meanwhile, we had another fundraiser planned, this time in Wisconsin. Our friends Melanie, Stephanie, Dustin, Brad, and Elizabeth had organized it and this one was set up as a barbeque, reminiscent of our annual Big BBQ from our OC days. Jessica came up to stay with Bec and I got a weekend away. It was fantastic.

Again, I was amazed by how much work our friends had done to support us. It felt amazing to not worry that there was some major medical risk even though I was away from Rebecca. Between insane amounts of pulled pork, great raffles, and a lot of beer, it was a blast. I got to tell the same stories to new people and lose my voice talking too loud which was my thing. The event flew by, was a huge success, and I headed back to our quiet apartment life.

During this time, I was feeling particularly unmotivated. I had planned to do all sorts of things once Rebecca got out of the hospital and was recovering. I bought a guitar that I was going to learn how to play. We were also near a nice running path and I was going to run every morning and lift every afternoon. I had found my old Rosetta Stone CDs and was going to finally finish my Spanish lessons. I would read several books and learn about the writing process. I would also have time to plan my business, whatever that was going to be.

This had not been a complete failure. I was doing my guitar lessons a couple of times a week. I was running and lifting but far from the two-a-days I had planned. I never even picked up the Spanish CDs and the reading and writing progressed, albeit slowly. Business plans had shifted from one idea to another which I would dig into long enough to either discount them or put them on a "potential" list.

Even though I would wake well before Rebecca, I spent a lot of time sort of waiting for her. While she was sleeping in the morning, I would sometimes read but I was always distracted, waiting to see when she would wake up and how she felt. It did not help that I had aches and pains from my rotator cuff and lower back. The first few hours of my day were dedicated to getting caffeinated and losing the pain. By then it was close to the time where Becca would wake and I would need to focus on getting her to start her treatments or eat.

When she got up, it didn't help that she wanted me to sit on the couch with her and watch a show. All she wanted to do was sleep on my lap while I played with her hair which helped to relax her. That sounded nice but after a morning of doing almost nothing, doing nothing together felt incredibly lazy.

She also seemed very down in the morning. I tried to counter this with coffee as quickly as possible but this only augmented the GERD (gastroesophageal reflux disease) issues she had. When I finally did get her talking, she would often talk about her job. She was depressed that she could not go back to work. Her job gave her a great sense of accomplishment. She excelled at it and supporting drug development trials made her feel like she was doing something of value.

The morning she opened up about it, she told me she had not slept much the night before. She was up thinking about how she could go back to work. Though we had spoken about it a few times before, I had never realized how important it remained. It struck me as simply too soon. At three months post-transplant, she had not fully healed and had a long way to go. I quietly questioned whether she would ever be healthy enough. Also, being awake for so few hours each day, even if she dedicated all of her non-eating, non-treatment hours to work, she would only be working part-time. She would not come close to matching her disability income, so it would cost us money for her to go back to work.

Meanwhile, our "new" house was not fully unpacked, particularly the office to which she had laid claim. The house was not decorated and we had boxes hidden in all of the nooks and crannies. After heading back there alone on so many nights, I wanted it to feel like a home. I had looked forward to doing the physical work and awarding her with a supervisory position.

If she returned to work, there was no halfway. It would become her top priority and like before, she would sacrifice eating, sleeping, and exercise to get a report submitted and maintain her metrics. Her words suggested that the reward was worth all that she would be giving up but her plan was based on her powering through it. I would not watch her work herself into the ground again.

We had already spoken about how it would consume almost all of our time together and it bothered me that she was so willing to sacrifice this for whatever satisfaction or accomplishment she drew from her work. I had sacrificed my career goals for her health, but I could not understand why she had so much trouble sacrificing her career for her own health, especially when that had been our plan for years. It was maddening.

We always knew that at some point she would be too sick to work. This was a driver for much of my career planning and aspirations, in part to take care of her financially. For over ten years, I had been working toward the goal of managing a business, leading a team, taking on new challenges and responsibilities. I may not have loved my job in the same way that Rebecca loved hers, but it meant a lot to me and I had devoted countless hours toward my achievements.

All of this changed on that New Year's Eve. I was not able to go back to work so as my vacation ticked away, my thought process had begun. I expected that I would be unemployed when applying to my next position and likely have to take a cut in pay. It would likely take longer to achieve the goal of being a GM and it was now unlikely that I could do so before I turned forty. I also had to consider that once I was a GM, the hours would only get longer.

I learned to be honest with myself that I was not ready to give that much of my time to a company while sacrificing time with my wife. We did not need to be together 24/7 but I was not ready to return to twelve-hour work days. Rebecca's desire to go back, even part-time, was the equivalent of those twelve-hour days.

Here I was re-evaluating a plan that I had for most of my adult life, while Becca was pushing back against a situation that we had expected. I had to rationalize that this same stubbornness was an attribute that got her through so many tough battles that year. It was central to her personality and therefore a big part of why she had managed to survive. That was at least some consolation.

We had been career focused for so long that work always seemed to hang over our heads. Before she was hospitalized, I was working long hours at a new job and Bec was fully occupied with either work or sleep. We would put in a few hours over the weekend and it was even rare if we fully enjoyed a vacation.

The day before Rebecca went on life support, we had both worked all day. When I called her at the end of the day to come by for a visit, she was worn out and planned to go to bed early. That conversation came very close to being the last one we ever had. It could have been our last opportunity to spend the day together and we spent it apart. I knew that there was a lesson there.

I thought about this many times as I sat in the hospital room as Rebecca lay there in a chemically induced coma. If your loved one has a disease like CF, you cannot leave your job every time they go in the hospital. There is a kind of routine that is almost comforting to know that each hospitalization is not of earth-shattering importance. So if most tune-ups were routine, how do you separate the critical ones?

I usually relied on either my own instincts or her telling me that she needed me there. I would otherwise try to be there whenever my work would allow. Even in retrospect, there was no way for me to tell that she would have gotten so much worse in one twenty-four-hour period. So if I should not leave work for every hospitalization and I had no way to predict the severity of each instance, then expecting us both to know when we should step away from work was essentially holding us to an impossible standard.

Perhaps the answer was in the big picture. How much time were we spending together, not just that day but that year, the past ten years, for our whole relationship? Was our relationship strong? Were there any major regrets? If we made time for each other, it did not matter that we did not make time every day. If we had a good relationship it did not matter if we got into an occasional argument. If we treated each other well, we had nothing to regret. If all of this was good, then maybe the point was that one event did not matter.

Of course we all want to leave things well and have the perfect last days with a loved one but that is not always possible. We should not beat ourselves up if it does not go perfectly as planned; that is not the purpose of a relationship.

Lesson 36: The point is not to have a beautiful moment with your loved one on that last day. The point is to have a beautiful relationship.

It is wonderful if you are lucky enough to do both but don't beat yourself up over an unfortunate final note. If Rebecca passed in January, I do not think I would have been plagued with regret because we had always made time together. Sure, in 2014 we were busier and more preoccupied but it was a decision we had weighed long before I had accepted the job, before we had purchased our house, and before Rebecca had petitioned her company to maintain employment in a new location. We had thought about this balance and we accepted the fact that we would have a busy year.

Work-life balance is not about balancing every day or every week, it is about a lifetime of balance. It is about taking the time to look at every tradeoff and consciously considering them in the decision. We had thought through these tradeoffs much more carefully because we knew the stakes. I was often the one pulling the reins in on Rebecca because I knew that balancing twenty years of overworking with twenty years of blissful retirement would not work out for us. There were few good things that CF brought to the equation...perspective and timeliness was among them.

CF also drove reflection. We were constantly benchmarking and comparing her current health status to her well-being from previous years. In high school, she ran cross country and had pulmonary function tests (PFTs) that were off-the-charts good. During college she once told me that she had lungs of a thirty-six-year-old. In her mid-thirties when she started on oxygen she reflected on previous years when it was completely unnecessary. Unfortunately, this reflection was typically a comparison to a healthier time. As we approached October, we were faced with a huge reminder of Rebecca's downturn. It all started on that nice weekend away in the mountains.

October 4, 2015: Blog Post

A year ago today…

…we walked into an urgent care clinic in Granby, CO. Rebecca's O_2 saturation (sats) was 52% and the nurse could not believe that she was able to stand there in front of her. After some initial tests, they worried she could be septic and suggested we take her by ambulance to Denver. Our quick weekend away with friends turned out to be a major turning point in Rebecca's health.

While we sat there waiting for the doctor's recommendation, Becca sent me on a mission to get her a snack. I figured I would get her the most joyous snack in the vending machine…the Almond JOY. Surprisingly, joy was not an emotion I felt in the moment pictured below. After pumping in $2 for a $1 bar, I walked away with the prize.

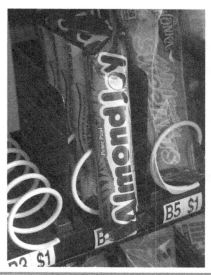

Not surprisingly, Rebecca was not in the mood for any Almond JOY by the time I returned. I carried that $2 candy bar with me for the 90 mile ambulance ride as I texted her mom and sister to keep them in the loop.

Her sats had never dropped that low. I had never seen her that sick. At the time, our major concern was sepsis, a life threatening condition caused by the body's response to an infection.

Not long after arriving in Denver, we found out that Rebecca was not septic. It was time to celebrate…Almond JOY time. Though we still faced the reality of her failing lungs, there was a huge feeling of relief

It was a major turning point in our mindset. In the course of one day, the lung transplant discussion became less frightening…by comparison. Our short weekend in the mountains quickly changed to a week in the hospital as we waited for her condition to improve enough so that she could fly home on settings that a portable oxygen concentrator could support. From then on, she took a wheelchair through the airports and always had O_2 with her.

It was also a major turning point for her health. She switched to supplemental oxygen almost 24 hours a day as her lung function dropped significantly. We later learned that she had experienced heart failure on the right side. Her heart needed to work so much harder because her lungs were slowly failing.

What I learned from that situation was that you need to celebrate good news even when there's bad news on the horizon and that keeping a positive attitude is a reminder of why recovering is so important…

I never did get my extra dollar back for that Almond JOY but we got our $2 worth!

This was the first time we could do a year over year comparison of her health and say that things were actually better. With her extended sleeping hours and painful mornings, it was important to focus on the improvements by remembering how far she had come.

Her cats, on the other hand, were dealing with emotions that I did NOT understand. Sometimes these emotions would manifest themselves by the cats urinating into the clean laundry basket while other times a simple shit by my pillow would do the trick. Most of these emotions hit them around 4 a.m. when they would sprint around the apartment, meowing loudly, and scratching our couch. Since our apartment complex did not allow cats, this presented a bit of a problem. I would try to whisper-yell at them, "SHUT UP, CATS! STOP THAT!"

Once that failed, I would fire the water bottle in the air as a warning shot. This would quiet them down long enough for me to start to doze off before they started up again. I tried separating them, putting them together in a room, giving them free reign, locking them in our room...nothing worked. Finally, my mom sent us a toy with a motorized arm that, once activated, distracted their little cat minds from being horrible.

Meanwhile, Rebecca was still in a little bit of a funk, primarily because of her continued pain and fatigue, but partially because of her desire to return to work. I needed to find a way to lift her spirits. New tour dates for her favorite singer, Grace Potter, were released and I was excited that she was coming to Pittsburgh. We had listened to her music for years and I played it in Becca's hospital room as something familiar to battle her delirium. I had a little surprise for her...

September 7, 2015 Blog Post:

Grace Potter and a Delirious Beccalicious

"The day turns into night, turns into day, and I'm still delirious" is part of the chorus for a song on Grace Potter's new album, "Midnight". Bec quickly took a liking to it…though it's a song about partying, we joked about the ICU delirium she suffered from occasionally this year in the hospital. Part of the reason it affects people is that there's not much of a distinction between day and night and you often lose track of time.

To combat ICU delirium, they say to have familiar faces around, have a window nearby, and play familiar music. We listened to this advice and the music we played most often in Becca's hospital room was Grace Potter. Even while she was sedated and intubated during January, we felt it would help keep a positive mood in her room. It was then that I started an email exchange with Grace's management that led to a sweet little surprise last night. The email was titled "Beccalicious and Grace Potter."

We arrived at the Grace Potter concert an hour before the doors opened so we could secure a good spot near the stage. At the time I didn't know if my request for a meet and greet would pay off and I thought it was unlikely. I had kept her manager up to speed with Becca's condition and let him know when we would be attending a show but I had not heard back in a while. I checked my email in a blind hope that I would have a new response to our exchange and I have to say, I was surprised when I saw it. It was short and sweet and included "…might be able to make this work tonight." I sent him my number and waited for a call…

Like a secret agent, I stepped away when I saw the call come in from the tour manager. I received instructions to get her to the double doors left of the stage at

8:45. I was on it! I returned to Bec and played off coolly that it was the blood donation center calling. We had it all under control. I only started to get nervous at about 8:20 when Bec had to leave our spot to potentially throw up as her nausea often strikes at the least opportune times.

Hoping her Ondansetron (pronounced 'on Dance-a-tron') would kick in quickly and wouldn't cause us to miss this opportunity, I asked our new friends next to us if they could hold our spots while we went backstage. They were more than happy to oblige.

Luckily, Bec came back in time and we were off to the double doors for our meet and greet. She didn't know why I was pulling her over there but she came along with no fuss. As we waited near the area, I told her that I was trying to score some seats in case she got tired. She bought it long enough for the tour manager to come out and get us. He sat us in a cafeteria while we waited and that was when he said "she" would be ready soon. I could watch the realization slowly sink in that we were getting more than a couple of seats...

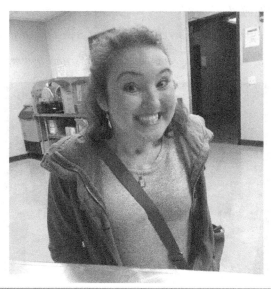

We sat there with anticipation building until the tour manager came to get us and bring us to a bench outside of her changing room. Before we knew it, Grace came out with a huge smile and gave Becca a big hug. She was thrilled! I got a hug too but not before Bec complemented her on her "gams."

333

We chatted for longer than I expected and I got to tell her the story of our inside joke with "Delirious." Bec was surprised that Grace knew her story and loved every second of the meet and greet.

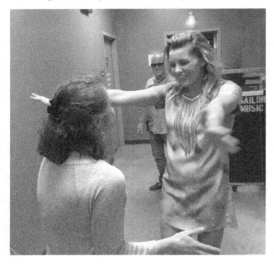

After a group shot it was time for the show. Grace said she would find us in the audience and she did.

I only regretted the fact that I didn't tell her how I had bought a guitar during her time in the hospital, mastered the G chord, and (given enough time) could play the D chord in succession. I am pretty sure that she may have found a spot for me in her band right then and there. In any case, I will be sure to put that in the thank you note.

We made it back to our spot up front that our friends had saved and watched an awesome show. During which, she gave Bec a pic and even dedicated a song to her…Delirious. Because of my amazing observational skills and lightning fast reflexes, I was able to catch some of this on video however a lack of acceptable formats and patience prevents me from figuring out how to post them here just yet…

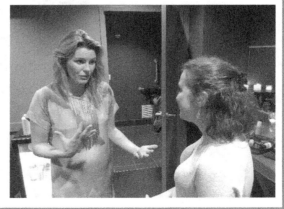

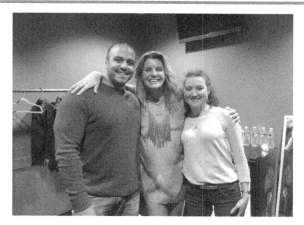

I'll try to post the videos on "The Rebecca Martello Poole Lung Transplant Journey" Facebook page.

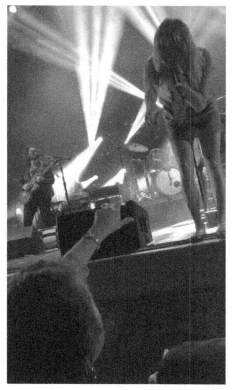

BEST. CONCERT. EVER.

CHAPTER 25

Not so Fast

I was incredibly confident going into the four-month bronch. Improvement had come consistently and relatively quickly since the transplant. Her recent PFTs had climbed to 85 percent while her weight had increased into the recommended range. Aside from the task of having to hold her pocketbook (that did not entirely match my shoes) I was feeling pretty good about the day.

As expected, the bronch was quick and the pulmonologist came out to tell me that everything looked great. She had taken some biopsies but those results would not be back for a few days. Becca would be tired from the general anesthetic and it would take twenty-four to forty-eight hours to work its way out of her system. I knew the drill, a couple of days of binge watching on the couch and she would be as good as new. We were going into the weekend and I had a fantastic excuse to be lazy. Bec would ask me to stay on the couch with her and I could use that request to justify not doing all of the things I should probably be doing. As the third and fourth day after the procedure passed, I was surprised to see that she was still so tired. Again, I chalked it up to Rebecca's unsurpassed ability to sleep.

By Monday I started to get a little concerned. Aside from

getting up for food and to do her breathing treatments, she laid down all day long. I suggested calling her post-transplant coordinator but she shrugged it off as unnecessary.

I finally mustered the motivation to get to the gym for a cardio kickboxing class that I had been meaning to check out. This is one of the few types of group classes I can take without looking like a goon. There is not much worse than going to a class where they are doing 80s-style aerobics moves, so I had determined that kickboxing was the safest. The only other box I was hoping to check was a second dude showing up for the class. Just before it started, a guy walked into the class and I was ready to go.

Despite its name, there was little kicking and very few moves that resembled any type of fighting. When the teacher started a move where you throw both hands up and over your head to the beat, I realized that things had gone horribly wrong. I had selected a position near the door so I could potentially escape if necessary, but the class was too small for me to escape unnoticed. So I spent the whole time trying to modify the moves so I could retain a shred of my masculinity. When the class was over, I was out, like the trash on a Thursday!

I got home ready to tell Bec my traumatic story and she stopped me with her first comment. "My coordinator called and I have acute rejection." Not much had recently taken me off guard, but this certainly did. She said she would have to go in for three days for infused steroids. I was glad that there seemed to be a standard treatment and I tried to let that comfort me. I reminded Rebecca that rejection was common and that it should be a simple fix. I wished I could have spoken with the coordinator but I had been too busy getting my jazzercise on.

I had become accustomed to talking to the doctors, having time to make sense of things, and then being able to present it to Rebecca in a way that would focus on the plan of action rather than the circumstance. Not only was I not there to "spin" the news, she had to digest it by herself for a half hour. I had so many questions but she did not have the answers to many of them. When would we have to follow up? How soon would we know if the rejection was gone? What was the probability it could be eliminated? I also wanted to know if I should continue to plan our move back to Cincinnati. She would be in the hospital through Thursday and our lease was up on Saturday. There was not much room for error or complications.

They would try to find a room for her the next morning but they would not succeed until the next night. We spent the day on the couch; this time it had a different feel. There was a sense of worry and dread as we sat there in the silence. She kept telling me, "I don't WANT to go back in." There was nothing I could say to ease her worry so I just tried to be positive. I told her how much better this visit would be compared to her last stay. She would be able to get up and walk around. She could use a regular toilet without any help. She had her voice back too. Plus, it was only for three days.

It was a long day. After going in once, then coming home because the available bed was not on the right floor, they called back when they had one ready. We got her settled and did some smooth talking to ensure her first treatment came that night. We were still on schedule.

The next day, she was in a bad mood. She was unhappy that she was back in the hospital and she was exhausted from being woken up every hour for a blood sugar check. She just wanted to be home. I reminded her that not only would she be out of the hospital, but she would be in our real home in less than a week.

We learned that some of her sleepiness from the past days could be due to the rejection. It was comforting to know that we had a plausible explanation for her increased sleep requirements. A follow-up bronch would be timed for two to three weeks after her steroid treatment concluded. This would tell us if the rejection had been eliminated. I went home that night feeling comforted that we were heading in the right direction.

The next morning, I was going to do some errands while Becca slept and she was going to text me when I should come in. I got started cancelling autopay for our rent, cable, internet, and electric. I did a little packing as well. My dad was due to arrive that night and Becca would come home the next day.

At almost 5 p.m., after not hearing from her, I texted her with no response. Finally, I called her and she said she was tired and felt horrible. She had a fever of 100.9°F and they were taking blood for some tests. We decided I would wait at home for my dad and continue packing.

It was not until the next morning that I saw her text from 1:26 a.m. stating they were transferring her to the MICU. Her blood pressure kept dropping and they were starting her on antibiotics. She would have to stay for the weekend. I convinced myself not to worry because there was no mention of her O_2 sats and she would be on antibiotics soon.

With my father up from Florida and a one-week extension on our apartment, I felt I had a handle on things. However, on our drive there, I got a call from *her* phone but it was the doctor's voice on the other end. I instantly flashed back to the last time this had happened...on New Year's Eve. Her message was the same; Rebecca had pneumonia and they needed to intubate her. What had gone so wrong?!

I walked in the room to what looked like a recap of New Year's Eve. They told me that she likely aspirated (refluxed into her lungs) and that was why she was having so much trouble breathing and (now) maintaining her O_2 levels. This is an added risk with transplant patients because it can increase the chance of rejection. However, that was not the immediate concern.

GERD was the cause of her pneumonia and subsequent intubation because the sphincter between her esophagus and stomach was not fully closing. This allowed stomach contents to flow upward into the esophagus and overflow into her lungs. This type of aspiration—called silent aspiration—was dangerous because we were completely unaware it was occurring (since it was unrelated to problems swallowing).

I stayed in the room as long as I could before the intubation procedure. I told her I loved her then we said our good-byes but I was able to hear her response this time—"I love you, too." I had no energy to call the entire family but they were at a point when all of them would understand the text update I sent and they knew they could call me with questions. They also knew about everything I was explaining. Unfortunately, it was not our first rodeo.

Initial feedback I received from the medical team was that she might be extubated in a day or so. I was REALLY hoping that was the case but knew that our Rebecca liked to make things complicated. The next doctor spoke with a much more concerned tone. He said that they were treating her for septic shock. Her blood pressure dropping was the result of the tone in her veins "relaxing" and potentially not bringing enough blood back to the heart to pump. She would get medication for this along with the antibiotics to fight the pneumonia. He pointed out that she was immunosuppressed from her transplant medications and that recovery would be a tougher challenge than it would be for a normal healthy person. Perhaps it would be a longer road than we had anticipated.

I wondered how she could have taken such a quick downturn. She had been doing so well on all accounts just a few days earlier and now we were talking about sepsis. In some respects, it felt like we were right back to where we were in January. It was so discouraging to see. There she was again, sedated, on a ventilator, a tube down her throat, and her hands secured to the bed. It was a sight I had hoped I would never see again. It was certainly one that I did not expect to see that year. I did what I knew to do...I sat by the bed, spoke to her, sang "The Beccalicious Song," and squeezed her hand three times so she knew I loved her. That was all I could do.

Though it was hard to see her wake up and start to kick, I did have a sort of numbness to everything. My mask was not needing replacement due to tears and snot as it did on New Year's Eve so I felt I was doing as well as I could be.

I recognized the next doctor to stop in. He was the same one who I spoke to the previous time she was intubated. He told me her white blood cell (WBC) count was low and he was going to give her Neupogen to bring it up. I suspected "low"" was an understatement and dug deeper to find out that it was 500 when it should be 5,000 wbc/mcL. He told me that they already started the treatment and that the backup plan was ECMO. At a point when I felt I could not be surprised, THAT was a surprise...ECMO?!?

I remembered her darkest days on ECMO when her spirits had dropped to their lowest point. I had to remind myself that I could not focus on something that might not happen. It continued to creep back into my thoughts and I continued to try to push it out.

As we left that night, I walked down the same hallway where she did so much of her post-transplant PT. It seemed like so long ago but it had only been a few months. Foremost on my mind was the contrast between then and now. I remember walking down that hallway to Rebecca's room so incredibly optimistic, knowing that she was getting stronger every day with her new lungs and her discharge pending. That same hallway now felt entirely different.

The best thing I could focus on was my plan of action. I needed a new, earlier schedule so I could be there during rounds. I also had to undo my plans from the previous day. I re-forwarded my mail back to Pittsburgh and then cancelled my cancellations for internet, cable, and electric. I also called my apartment and was able to get a one month extension. There was no way her team of doctors would want her leaving the state anytime soon, even if she had a major turnaround the next day.

Beyond that, I reminded myself of what was going our way. Had this illness hit a few days later, we could have been out of state and her transplant doctors would not have been there for the original diagnosis and treatment plan. We would have likely needed to arrange for a medical transport back to UPMC. I would have needed to reserve a hotel and not have the comfort or affordability of my apartment. My father would also not be there with me. It was important to recognize that we were fortunate, and to be thankful.

The next day I returned to more of the same. I was told to expect three to five days before the antibiotics kicked in. She had cultured a staph infection and they were able to refine her antibiotics. Her white count was still low but all other indications pointed toward improvement.

Previously she had told me that she remembered nothing from January when she was in the same state. The sedation prevented her from remembering all that had occurred, which was a nice relief to me before, and an even better one now. She would not remember any of this. So, when I saw her kick her legs or pull her arms, I decided that I was not going to harbor those same worries. Being concerned about her condition rather than how she looked made it easier to look at her in the bed again. I knew that by all meaningful measures, she was out.

This comforted me into the next day because she was a little more riled up when I came in. As I spoke with the doctors, they all seemed to feel she was headed in the right direction. I continued to worry about her white count but was consoled by the fact that she was no longer in septic shock. They explained that it wasn't severe and that it resolved quickly. At least I had something positive to hold onto. Unfortunately, that news was not going to cheer anyone else up because I had not told anyone that she was suffering from sepsis.

As various caregivers came in to talk with us over the course of the day, two key doctors (the ICU fellow and pulmonologist) told me that they thought we might be able to extubate her the next day. She could be off the ventilator that quickly! This would be a fantastic departure from a January repeat and I let myself get excited about this idea. I knew that she would do better if she was awake and had the ability to cough up the junk that still resided in her lungs. She would also be one step closer to getting some fuel in her system.

She had not received any tube feeds since coming to the ICU because they did not want her to aspirate again. It almost seemed like I was watching her get thinner as she lay there on her hospital bed. Her hands were getting puffy again and her legs looked smaller to me. I knew how much atrophy she experienced the last time and she was getting tube feeds then. Here she lay without them and the time was ticking away. She needed to get extubated!

On morning four in the ICU the RT told me that Becca had been on weaning mode twice now and each time her respiratory rate climbed and she was switched back to pressure support. As they explained this, I remembered the sedation reductions and weaning times in Cincinnati and I was instantly convinced that this was related to her anxiety. This gave me a plan. I needed to convince everyone that her anxiety was causing her elevated respiratory rate and not any other kind of weakness or lack of endurance. When the RT came back to wean her again, Becca's respiratory rate immediately climbed from 22 to 40 breaths per minute and she was ready to stop it. I smooth talked her into waiting but I knew she would be back soon.

I proceeded to tell every caregiver that came near her. As the day went on, they wanted to test the waters. They turned off her propofol, because she needed to be somewhat awake. Her eyes began to open and she was visibly upset. She was hard to understand but was motioning with her right arm in a way that highlighted the restraints. I told her that they needed to stay on, and I saw her eyes tearing up. She was so upset and confused that all I wanted to do was to hug her. However, I resisted because she had little interest in hugging right then.

The fellow and attending came in to asses her readiness for extubation. They seemed to be on the fence but leaning toward going through with it. Unfortunately they were asking her if she wanted it. No one could understand what she kept trying to say but then she would shake her head *no*. It appeared that she did not want the tube out but I knew better. She was trying to tell us something that we would probably never understand...maybe about the humidity in the room...

I told them that she was still pretty out of it and that I could approve of any procedure if they needed that. We gave her a pen and paper and she drew some fantastic scribbles for us. The whole time I was just hoping for a single nod *yes* then I could play it up and we could get this thing moving. Finally, after about five minutes of scribbling, they asked her again and she said *yes*. Whether she knew what the hell they were talking about did not matter to me one bit...she was getting extubated!

She did not want me to leave the room so I was fortunate enough to get a front row seat. It was a much better show than a trach change but I would still not recommend it. They pulled the tube out and she started coughing hard. She coughed up quite a bit and her cough continued to sound clearer. I settled in for an interesting afternoon of Sedation Becca.

First she asked for her toothbrush. She was very upset with me when she realized I did not have any toothpaste for her but I managed to convince her to brush with water. She had a little trouble getting the toothbrush to her mouth so I took over while she only protested a little. Then, she was back to the toothpaste topic as she asked me to get the nurse. We were able to get some cleaning liquid which she ultimately came to accept.

The next topic was thirst. I had to be the bearer of bad news telling her that she could not drink but we got the nurse to get us some wet sponges. It was enough. During one of her refills however, she informed me...

"This holy water makes my back hurt."

"So, this is holy water and it's causing your back pain?"

"Yes. The holy water hurts my back," she told me with

certainty.

Of course it bothered me that her back hurt but I loved how she skipped past all of the reasoning and jumped right to the conclusion. I could not decide what was funnier, the fact that she knew it was holy water, or the certainty with which she determined that it caused her back pain. There was not much I could say but, "I'm sorry, dear," and hope she nodded off.

The next morning, she looked stronger and more alert. She was also more concerned and asked how her dad was doing. She was upset because she had dreamt he had been shot. It took a lot of convincing to let her know that he was fine. I even lied and told her that we had just spoken. That seemed to do the trick.

Much like Neo in *The Matrix*, she could not yet tell reality from the dream world. Unfortunately, her dreams were more like nightmares so not surprisingly, she seemed very depressed. After all of the work she had put in to move forward, she had a pretty big setback. I hoped that it was her dream that depressed her and not reality.

She was finally starting to gain confidence in her new lungs and now she had a rejection scare, an aspiration incident, and was intubated for days. That would be a letdown for anyone, especially after a tough year like this had been.

I liked to "lead the witness," so as we sat down I asked if she was doing well. Waiting for a simple *yes*, I received another confusing response...

"I was, until Timmy shot the organist!"

"Timmy shot the organist?"

"He did," she confirmed. I could see that she was quite displeased with Timmy.

"Was it an organist in a church?"

"Yes."

"Was it your stepbrother Timmy or nephew Timmy?"

"It was my brother...that son of a bitch!" she snarled like a gun slinger in the Old West. When she started to get upset, I realized I had to stop prodding her for more of the story and just tell her the truth.

"Timmy didn't shoot the organist, Bec. Nobody shot anyone. You're still a little delirious from all of the meds and that was all a dream..."

Over the next days as she became more alert, I assumed she was mostly back to reality. Aside from getting annoyed at me because she had dreamt I told her we were in Cincinnati, she was mostly on track.

I brought up her comment on the holy water hurting her back and I expected that she would either laugh or not remember it at all. Straight-faced, she confirmed it with passion. "That holy water sucked. It tasted awful!" She explained that the nurse-nuns were supposed to reconstitute her meds with holy water but that her favorite nurse-nuns would use sterile water. She planned to ask my mom why the holy water was pink and reiterated, "Every time I got it, it hurt my back."

It was during that conversation that I learned about how comprehensive Becca's delusion had been. She thought we had been in a convent and it was near our house in northern Kentucky. The nurses there were also nuns. They could only drink holy water and even made their tea from it. She continued to explain to me that her stepbrother Timmy came in pretending to be hurt so he could get narcotics. He then went on a shooting spree and shot the organist, her father, and tried to shoot her but she was wearing his motorcycle helmet that protected her.

It must have been awful, not being able to fully wake up from this terrible dream. Imagining these horrible scenarios and the people she loved being so involved. But...a helmet protected her? I saw all of the seriousness that Recovering Becca had in her wide-open eyes, and then I imagined her with a big, round, bulletproof, helmet. I bet it was red. It would take a few days to fully convince her that these nightmares were not real.

She was quite annoyed at me when she found out that we were in Pittsburgh because apparently it was Dream Ray who told her we were near our house. This dream version of me resulted in real me getting some serious side eye action from our favorite patient.

It was not long before her nausea returned. By this point, I was deathly afraid of it, partially because of the aspiration that had recently rained on our recovery parade. As each instance came and went, I got a little less anxious about it. The real issue was reflux. I reasoned that it took four months before GERD had caused an issue, and that was starting from the transplant date. Reflux aspiration was a major concern, but we probably had enough time to resolve it before it struck again. The important thing was that she was recovering from this and we were going to fix the underlying cause.

We decided to get a work up for a surgery called Nissen

fundoplication. This would tighten the sphincter between her stomach and esophagus and prevent reflux from happening. This was no minor procedure and there were several variations, so the work up was an important step in determining the specifics of what was to be done.

We also learned that all of her medications for GERD, like antacids and drugs like Pepcid, only reduced the acidity of her stomach acids, thereby reducing her pain. Stomach fluid was still getting into her esophagus, potentially causing aspirations whether she felt it or not. This information only made the situation more worrisome and urgent.

As much as I worried about the next time, I knew that all we could do was focus on one battle at a time. Over the next few days, she improved clinically; she looked and appeared better by evaluation. Unfortunately, her X-rays kept getting worse. We needed to get her up and walking to cough a bunch of that junk out. One day, when the doctors rounded, they told her that if she did not get up and start moving, she could end up in the ICU again.

Since waking up from this incident, Rebecca was even more down than normal. She would sit there and look off to the side. She did not want to watch TV nor did she have much to say. She was just miserable. It was incredibly discouraging to take these steps back after all of her improvements. Hell, she was two weeks into her "Couch to 5K" program and had planned to run a race in the spring. Now here she was, suddenly stuck in a hospital bed with major stomach issues, struggling to breath, and notably weaker than just a week before.

During rounds, Rebecca constantly pressed her doctors about leaving and going home. I knew she would be happier there but I also knew that she would not have an ICU downstairs or doctors checking on her daily. It would be on me to catch the signs of an aspiration if it happened and she would not have constant monitoring of her O_2 levels. Her body often decided to have problems in the middle of the night. She could have an incident that I might sleep through, or worse, we might not decide to go into the hospital until it was too late. Returning home was not something I wanted to rush.

I did, however, use it as motivation for her. If we could get walking and cough up more of the junk in her lungs, then her X-rays would start improving and she could get out of there. It seemed to work but it was a reminder to her that she had lost a lot of strength. I had to support her quite a bit during our first walk but she rebounded quickly. By the following Monday, just short of two weeks in the hospital, she was discharged. Not only was she out of the hospital, but after her follow up bronchoscopy, she was cleared to move back home in time for Thanksgiving. It could not have worked out better. Well...no aspiration pneumonia would have been better but why split hairs?

After seeing Rebecca so down, day after day, then seeing her sink lower during this hospitalization, my main goal was lifting and maintaining her spirits. I looked forward to getting discharged from the hospital and continued physical recovery.

Brenda, who had been back in Idaho since shortly after the transplant, would periodically get frustrated by Rebecca's infrequent calls and lay guilt on her. I hated to see Bec constantly apologizing for her failure to keep in touch when she had so much else to deal with.

This pressure was especially frustrating from someone who had not sent a single get well card that year…communication when it counted.

Jessica suggested that Brenda blamed me for their infrequent communication, as if I was deleting messages or hiding Becca's phone from her. I saw Brenda blame Becca and even texted her stating that Bec knew her name and number, and that Brenda had screenshots of the times she had called and proof that Rebecca had not called her back. These angry texts made me want to tell her to back off, that this was not about her, and that it did not help Rebecca.

Deep down, I knew that this would not motivate her to change. I decided to hold off and that another confrontation should only take place after all other tactics were employed. So an expertly written, thinly veiled Facebook post about Rebecca's medical struggles and lack of free time to return calls would have to suffice. It would have been easier to call and scold her since I felt I had nothing to lose, but it was not the best way.

Lesson 37: Even after a relationship is damaged, continue to look for diplomatic routes to resolve issues. Conflict should remain a last resort.

CHAPTER 26

You *Can* Go Home Again

When Thanksgiving arrived it served as the best welcome home party we could imagine. Between Jessica's family, Pete, and my dad, we had a full house. There was a quiet appreciation in the air that we could gather together as we did every year.

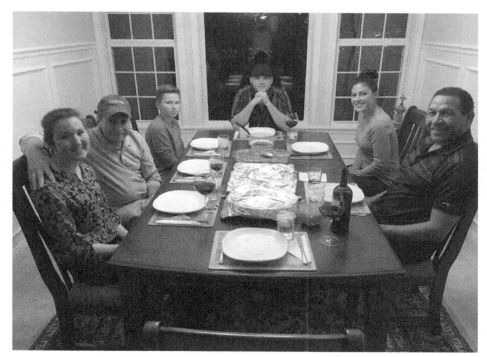

Clockwise: Rebecca, Pete, Cole, Trey, Jessica, Ray (Sr.)

November 26, 2015: Facebook post

We started this year with Rebecca on a ventilator. In the picture below, she had woken up for a second and asked me to take her picture so she would know what she looked like. Right afterwards, she gave me this double-thumbs-up.

Months later, after a half year on a ventilator, multiple emergency ICU visits, a mechanical lung (ECMO), sepsis, heart issues, and way too much more...she's up and running with plans to do a 5k in the spring. Now she has no rejection, no infection, the best lung function test in years, and a house full of family.

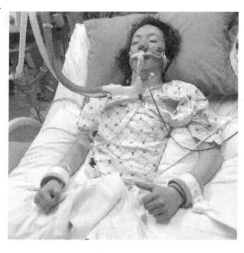

We have a lot to be thankful for this year and we couldn't expect to be doing any better than we are today.

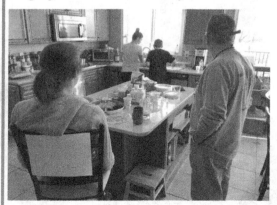

For today, the biggest challenge is keeping her in her 'suggestion' chair so she doesn't overdo it. Actually...that is a REAL challenge. Happy Thanksgiving!

We even identified Rebecca's chair with a sign: Director's Chair AKA Suggestion Seat => Rebecca's.

December brought some relaxing time at home. We were able to settle in a bit more and got to see Meg again. It was such a drastic change since the last visit that concluded in the CTICU with Rebecca on ECMO.

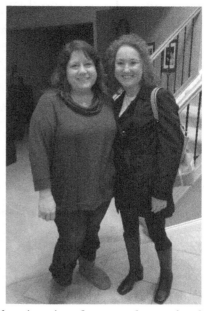

Another bout of pneumonia came along with December, likely from another silent aspiration. A temperature of 103.9°F had us racing off to the ER. She ended up in the ICU again, but was not intubated and the situation fortunately resolved with a quick round of antibiotics.

During her last night in the hospital, she recognized her RT; it was the lady who had brought her down to the MICU on New Year's Eve. This was the person she brought up for weeks after waking up at the Drake Center who had told her, "You don't have to work so hard," and was so nice to her. To me, that was what a caregiver should be…someone who made an impact by not only their actions, but their words. We spoke about a victory tour through all of the hospital wings where she had spent time; this seemed to be the perfect start.

She was soon well enough to make the journey to Connecticut for Christmas and New Year's Eve and the holidays were a stark contrast to the year before.

December 31, 2015 Blog Post:

A New Year for Bec…

It's easy to get a little reflective on New Year's Eve but this one in particular marks a major milestone for us. A year ago today, on New Year's Eve morning, I received a phone call from the hospital with an ICU doctor on the other line. He told me that Rebecca was not able to maintain her oxygen saturation levels even with 15 liters pumping through the canula. He stumbled through his words as he tried to explain the seriousness of the situation and that Rebecca was on BiPAP in the MICU…whatever that meant. I raced through the house doing a whole lot of nothing at a pretty fast pace until I reasoned with myself, "You don't have to perform surgery, you just have to show up."

I got to the hospital and she could barely talk. I would help to hold her mask so I could sponge a little water into her mouth every few minutes. That was the worst I had seen her. When they told us she would need to be placed on a ventilator, it was one of the first times I had ever seen her that afraid. I did not have to see that for long because they kicked me out of the room for the procedure. The doctor had to tell me that she had said "I love you," because her voice was too weak to be heard from the door.

I went downstairs and immediately called all of her family to bring them up to speed. It was a call that I always dreaded. I did not have many answers for them. I didn't know how long she would be sedated. I didn't know if this was normal. I didn't know if she would survive or how long she would have if she did. I had to make the calls anyway and do my best to keep everyone calm but informed. It was sometime near then that I set a goal for myself to keep them (and everyone else) updated on what was going on because she had so many people that cared about her.

Updates alone were not enough, the information needed to be accurate but not delivered in an alarming way. There wasn't much I could do in this crappy situation but I could do something that might be of a little value.

I returned to her room to see her looking so uncomfortable, sedated with the breathing tube down her throat, and all of a sudden it was just me. I had always expected that the two of us would be dealing with this together but that would not be the case. I remember the first time she coughed and wondering how she could get anything up around that tube. I remember the first time I heard the doctors say that she had "end stage CF," I remember asking a LOT of questions…some of which I didn't want the answers to…I remember way more details than I would like to from last New Year's Eve. I knew we were going to have our New Year's Eve in the hospital but I didn't realize that it was not going to be a celebration.

Rebecca woke up for long enough to find out that I was staying the night and spent 10 minutes trying to communicate with me that I should ask for a cot. She was sedated and intubated and worrying that my chair would suck. I supposed she also thought that I didn't have enough sense to ask for one myself. It seems that I really set the bar low in our previous 17 years together. It was okay though because they brought in a "nice" recliner for me to sleep on and I settled in for the long haul.

Reflecting on this past year, I could say it was pretty shitty. Between Becca being ventilated for six months, multiple pneumonias, a mechanical lung (ECMO), several discussions on her (unfavorable) odds, being turned down by five transplant centers, an emergency medical flight, and the end of my new job that had brought us to Cincy in the first place…I could definitely say "good riddance to a bad year!"

I'm not going to say that though… It was a tough year with some very bad parts but Rebecca started it unconscious and now she is awake. She was on a ventilator and ended the year with no need for supplemental oxygen. She was given "days to weeks" and a year later she is healthy and able to travel to Connecticut for Christmas. Last year this time, I was in a recliner sweating into a plastic gown and this year I'm in the living room while Bec takes a snoozer. 2015 was the year that Rebecca received her lung transplant and I'm going to call it a good year.

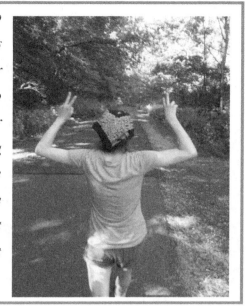

Central to how we made it through a tough year was to understand what power lay in interpreting the events. How we interpreted each situation influenced our perspective. We could look at January as simply an awful event or decide to be thankful that she beat the odds and lived through it.

We could have compared our challenging walks in February to a lifetime of strength and let it bring us down, or decide to compare them to January and be thankful she was awake and starting to build herself back up.

We could have viewed her rejection from five different transplant centers as five consecutive let downs or decide that their quick rejection allowed us to focus our time on the one center that would accept her.

We could have viewed ECMO as one of the worst health

declines of her lifetime but the resulting increase in her LAS was probably the reason why she received lungs in time to save her life.

These decisions for optimism were not one-time events. We had to decide every morning, every time we received an unfavorable diagnosis, and every time dread and pessimism creeped back in and we needed to remember what we had learned. There was no value in expecting the worst, nor was there value in stressing about things we could not change. If it were as easy as deciding what you would change if you could, I would have changed Rebecca's cystic fibrosis to a simple case of nymphomania and been done with it. For me, the serenity prayer said it best...

"God grant me the serenity to accept the things I cannot change,
Courage to change the things I can,
And wisdom to know the difference."
–Reinhold Niebuhr

Lesson 38: We do not have control of much but we can decide how to interpret events, how we want to view the world, and how to respond to the situations we find ourselves in.

If we let emotion overtake us and respond with our baser instincts, we can easily be left wrestling with guilt and regret. At the end of the day, we sit alone with our thoughts and memories. I want mine to be saturated with little victories, tons of laughs, and enough bright spots to outshine the dark.

EPILOGUE

I would have been ecstatic if you had told me in January 2015 that Rebecca would survive long enough to receive a lung transplant, so I was not about to let a longer-than-expected duration of uncertainty change my outlook. In 2015, Rebecca got her transplant and we *were* ecstatic—it was a good year.

As we moved into 2016, Rebecca did receive her stomach surgery. Delayed by pneumonia from another silent aspiration, the surgery resulted in a slew of complications. We initially thought that the surgery went well, then a few hours later, despite several blood transfusions, Rebecca's hemoglobin level continued to drop as her pain increased. She was bleeding internally. They raced off to do an exploratory surgery and found that the injury was in an unusual location. That night, after the surgery, they packed her open—they did not stitch her stomach closed but instead, covered the area with a clear plastic wrap. They were resigned that it could take several more surgeries before this was resolved. What should have been a three-day recovery stretched into two months. We again had instances where we worried for her life.

Over the next week, an abscess (pocket of fluid) developed in her abdomen and it cultured bacterial and fungal infections. While all of this happened, one of her new lungs partially collapsed. As she worked to recover, one of the new medications interacted with her anti-rejection medication causing a spike in tacrolimus levels to more than three times the target. This caused dehydration, kidney problems, and renewed concern with her heart. She was hospitalized twice more.

So what did she do? She got up and walked every day. We learned about a whole new set of concerns and did our best to deal with them. Thankfully it was enough. Though plagued with chest pain, stomach pain, weakness, and fatigue, she continues to push forward. Recovery is slow to progress but it progresses...one step back but two steps forward.

Like with everything else, she is battling back and recuperating like a rock star in rehab. The exceptional type of rock star that swallows more pills than you could imagine...but has never done blow.

LESSONS

1. Show up. (p. v)
2. Sometimes you have to trust your instincts, take a risk, and not focus on the worst that could happen. (p. 6)
3. Pick your battles but argue for the things that matter to you; it is better than holding a grudge. (p. 18)
4. Be thankful. (p. 53)
5. Ask a lot of questions and understand that you provide value even if you are not a medical expert. (p. 57)
6. Sometimes the best way to take care of someone else is to also take care of yourself. (p. 62)
7. Do not mourn for somebody that is alive. (p. 68)
8. Two steps forward and one step back is still an improvement. (p. 69)
9. Understand that things may not be as bad as they seem in the moment, give it time. (p. 76)
10. Do not take the worries of others onto your own shoulders. (p. 81)
11. There is nothing to be gained by comparing your pain with the intent to prove you are suffering more than others. You will only demonstrate that you lack empathy. (p. 97)
12. You have to celebrate the small victories because they add up to big victories. (p. 106)
13. Every day may not be a good day, but recognize that it is good to have that day. (p. 113)
14. Listen to what your loved ones want, even if it is not what you want for them. (p. 119)
15. Look for those things that bring joy and make them a part of your routine. (p. 124)
16. If you have the opportunity, laugh. (p. 125)
17. Writing down your thoughts can provide the impetus you need to move on. (p. 130)
18. A full night's sleep, whenever possible, must be a priority. (p. 133)
19. Make the time to maintain an exercise routine. (p. 135)
20. Plan for the worst, plan for the best, and plan for everything in between. (p. 143)
21. Be aware that when you get something off your chest it could end up on someone else's shoulders. Sometimes there is little value in setting the record straight. (p. 150)

22. There is no way to do everything for someone else all of the time. Try to recognize when and how you are needed the most. (p. 166)

23. People will respond to what you provide. If you want them to help you stay positive, show them how. (p. 179)

24. Don't be discouraged if you fall short. A failure today may be a blessing in disguise. (p. 182)

25. Try not to complain. Somebody always has it worse. Particularly, try not to complain to them. (p. 185)

26. Those who are not there do not need to know every detail in real time. Instead, just be present. (p. 196)

27. There's a thin line between telling nurses how to do their job and advocating for a loved one. Be aware of it, but know that you can dig your heels in. (p. 225)

28. Do not hesitate to ask for help. (p. 242)

29. The risk of being too hopeful then getting let down is a better option than expecting something miserable from the start. (p. 255)

30. If you feel like you're losing, keep fighting. You never know when something as simple as a single call can change everything. (p. 256)

31. Be aware of the mood and try to affect it in a positive way. (p. 264)

32. To stay motivated, maintain a vision of the future you want and try to imagine living it. (p.267)

33. When you realize that someone's disrespectful actions will continue, address them head-on. (p. 278)

34. Never underestimate the boost you can get from the support of others. (p. 314)

35. Mental recovery, like physical recovery, takes time and requires a surprising amount of patience. (p. 318)

36. The point is not to have a beautiful moment with your loved one on that last day. The point is to have a beautiful relationship. (p. 327)

37. Even after a relationship is damaged, continue to look for diplomatic routes to resolve issues. Conflict should remain a last resort. (p. 352)

38. We do not have control of much but we can decide how to interpret events, how we want to view the world, and how to respond to the situations we find ourselves in. (p. 359)

RESOURCES

To donate in honor of Rebecca visit:

> Cota.donorpages.com/PatientOnlineDonation/
> COTAforRebeccaP/

For additional details, photos, and other media covering Rebecca and Ray's journey visit:

> CFCornerman.com

To follow Ray's updates on social media and blog visit:

Twitter.com/CFCornerman	(@CFCornerman)
Instagram.com/CFCornerman	(@CFCornerman)
Facebook.com/CFCornerman	(@CFCornerman)
Facebook.com/RebeccaPooleCF	(@RebeccaPooleCF)
Raylpoole.wordpress.com	(Blog)

To learn more about Cystic Fibrosis visit:

Cystic Fibrosis Foundation:	CFF.org
Cystic Fibrosis Research Institute:	CFRI.org
U.S. Adult Cystic Fibrosis Assoc.:	CFroundtable.com

To learn more about organ donation and transplantation visit:

> Donatelife.net
>
> UNOS.org

ACKNOWLEDGMENTS

I would like to extend a special thanks to a few people...

To the donor and the donor's family, thank you for giving my wife the gift of life. We hope to thank you in person one day!

Rebecca Poole, my wicked smart wife. Thank you for believing in me, providing your valuable feedback, and even proofreading the book! The enduring courage you demonstrate inspires me every day. I am lucky to have you and am forever proud of you.

Rachel Saluzzi, you were there for me from the start with so many phone calls, cards, and visits. Even with managing a family and a full time job, you managed all of the fundraising efforts so that I could focus on Rebecca. You are amazing.

Louise Poole, Mom, between all of the cards and baked goods, you always had something in the mail and came out so often. And Rebecca says thank you for taking care of her cats.

Ray Poole, Dad, thanks for helping me move and staying in Pittsburgh from ECMO through transplant. I enjoyed celebrating every little victory together.

Scott Martello, thank you for the peace you bring to Bec and for being there when I needed to leave for the fundraiser.

Pete Bastien, thanks for so often asking how I was doing and for making it easier for Bec's sister to come out.

Jessica Bastien, you handled things like a champ and knew how to keep Becca smiling. Thanks for being there when we needed you.

Meghan Hughes, I always knew you'd do anything for us but a special thanks for being there each and every time you were needed, particularly when Rebecca was placed on ECMO.

ACKNOWLEDGMENTS CONT...

Karen Ang, thank you for helping me turn this book into a reality. Thanks for volunteering your time to edit the book and providing your expertise.

Melanie Romas, thanks for convincing me to write this book; it was more therapeutic than I could have realized. Perhaps I should have added that as a lesson— write a book.

Norman Eng, thanks for being there to talk to, to drag me to the movies, and to promise Rebecca bacon.

Thanks to the many visitors that traveled a long way to brighten our days.

Thanks to all of our friends and family that sent cards, gifts, snacks, and flowers. They always brought Rebecca up, even when I showed them to her the second, third, and fourth times.

Thanks to all of our friends that helped with the fundraisers in Connecticut and Wisconsin. Thanks to those who donated goods, those who donated their time, those who donated funds, and everyone who came out to support us. I was overwhelmed and humbled by the outpouring of support and cannot express how much I appreciated it.

Thanks to all of the staff at the University of Cincinnati Hospital, Daniel Drake Center, and University of Pittsburgh Medical Center who took such good care of Rebecca and literally kept her alive. Thanks to the doctors, nurses, RTs, PTs, aides, and social workers. A very special thanks to Dr. Patricia Joseph, Dr. Elsira Pina, Dr. Renee Hebbeler-Clark, Dr. Jonathan D'Cunha, Dr. Matthew Morrell, Dr. Joseph Pilewski, Kindra Stone, Ann Compton, Tennille Dotson Scott, Sue Goldmeier, Karen Montag, Pat Brown, Amanda Pearsol, and so many more!

ABOUT THE AUTHOR

Raymond Poole earned a BS degree in Mechanical and Materials Engineering from the University of Connecticut as well as an MBA from Indiana University. Throughout his career, he has worked in Operations, Engineering Management, and Marketing. Ray has earned a patent, a lean six-sigma certification, and has won two national championships in fighting.

Inspired by his wife Rebecca and her struggles with Cystic Fibrosis, Ray became involved with the Cystic Fibrosis Foundation and was named "Milwaukee's Finest" in 2013 in honor of his volunteerism and fundraising efforts. He became a member of the Wisconsin CFF Leadership Board and later won the 2014 Eaton Stover Volunteerism award.

He holds a third degree black belt in Tae Kwon Do and has trained and competed in several martial arts including Muay Thai and Jujitsu. In his spare time, Ray enjoys working on his cars, lifting weights, and entertaining friends and family. Ray does not enjoy running, but he does it anyway...like a boss.

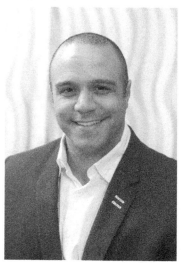

www.CFCornerman.com

Made in the USA
Monee, IL
16 October 2024

68073806R00213